Yoga for Pregnancy

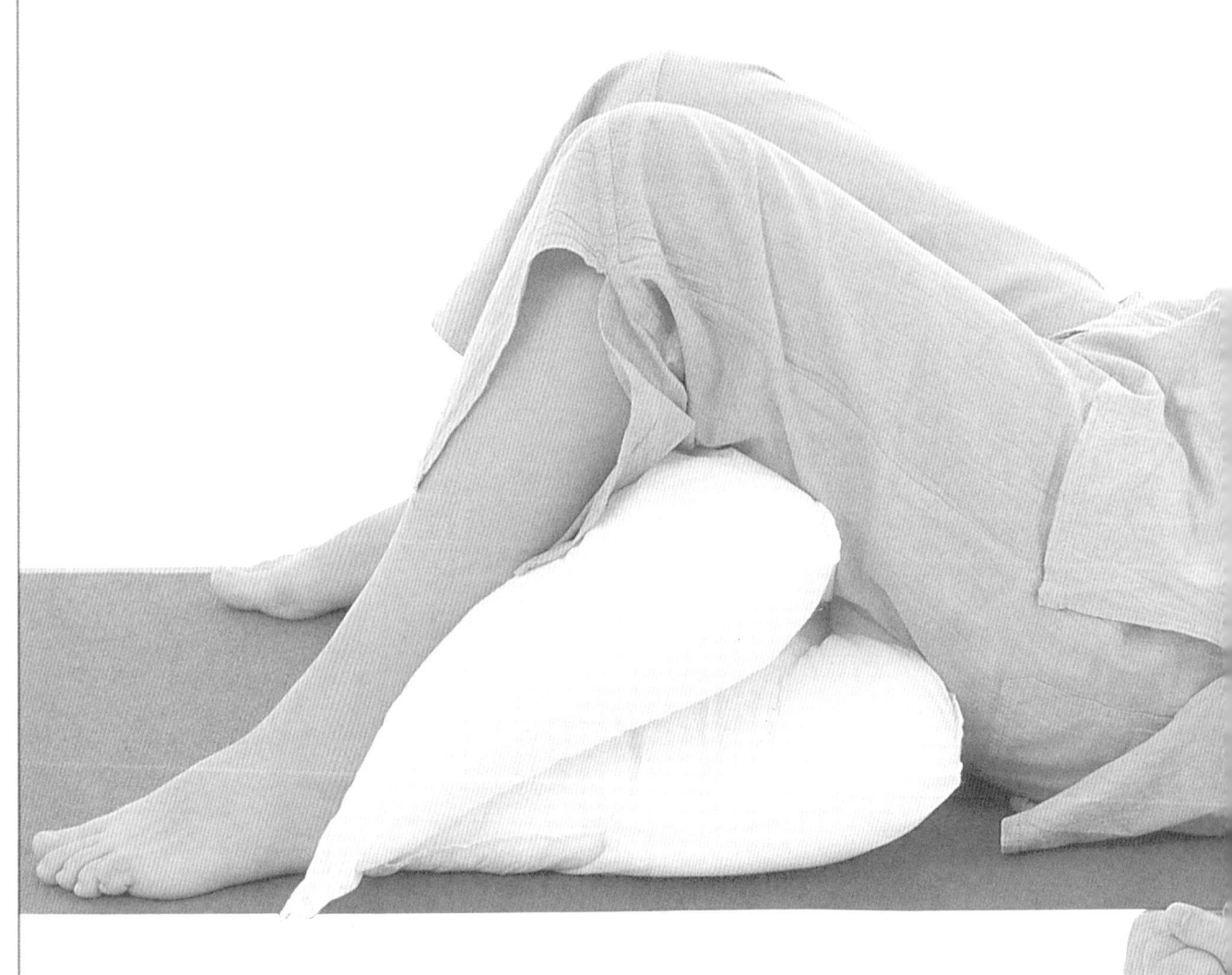

Yoga for Pregnancy

AMBER LAND

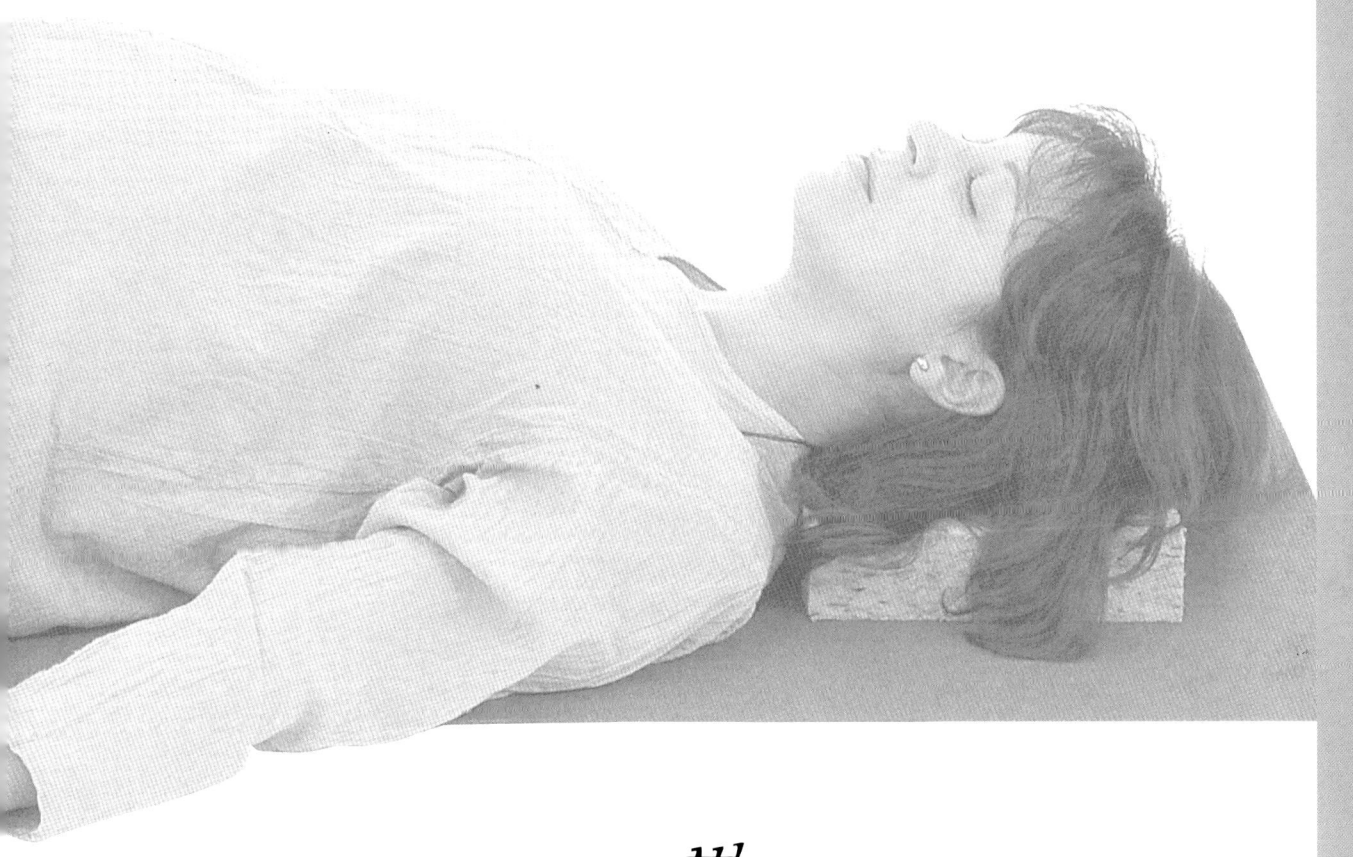

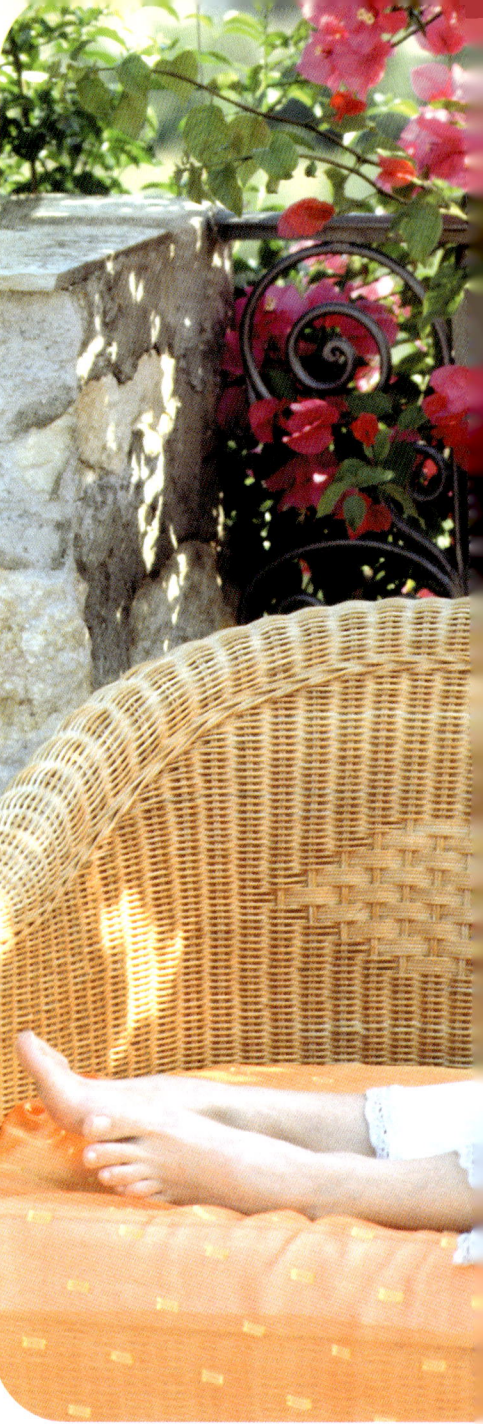

First published in 2003 by
New Holland Publishers
London • Cape Town • Sydney • Auckland
www.newhollandpublishers.com

86 Edgware Road
London W2 2EA
United Kingdom

80 McKenzie Street
Cape Town 8001
South Africa

14 Aquatic Drive
Frenchs Forest, NSW 2086
Australia

218 Lake Road
Northcote, Auckland
New Zealand

Copyright © 2003 New Holland Publishers (UK) Ltd
Copyright © 2003 in text: Amber Land
Copyright © 2003 in illustrations: New Holland Publishers (UK) Ltd
Copyright © 2003 in photographs: New Holland Image Library (NHIL) and individual photographers and/or their agents as listed on page 96.

All rights reserved. No part of this publication may be reproduced, stored in a retrieval system or transmitted, in any form or by any means, electronic, mechanical, photocopying, recording or otherwise, without the prior written permission of the publishers and copyright holders.

ISBN 1 84330 252 7 (HB), 1 84330 253 5 (PB)

Publisher: Mariëlle Renssen
Publishing Manager: Claudia Dos Santos
Managing Editor: Simon Pooley
Managing Art Editor: Richard MacArthur
Editor: Gill Gordon
Designer: Christelle Marais
Illustrator: Steven Felmore
Picture Researcher: Karla Kik
Production: Myrna Collins

Consultants: Simon Low, Sue Delft (UK)
Dr Peter Roos (South Africa)

Reproduction by Hirt & Carter (Cape) Pty Ltd
Printed and bound in Singapore by Craft Print International Limited

2 4 6 8 10 9 7 5 3 1

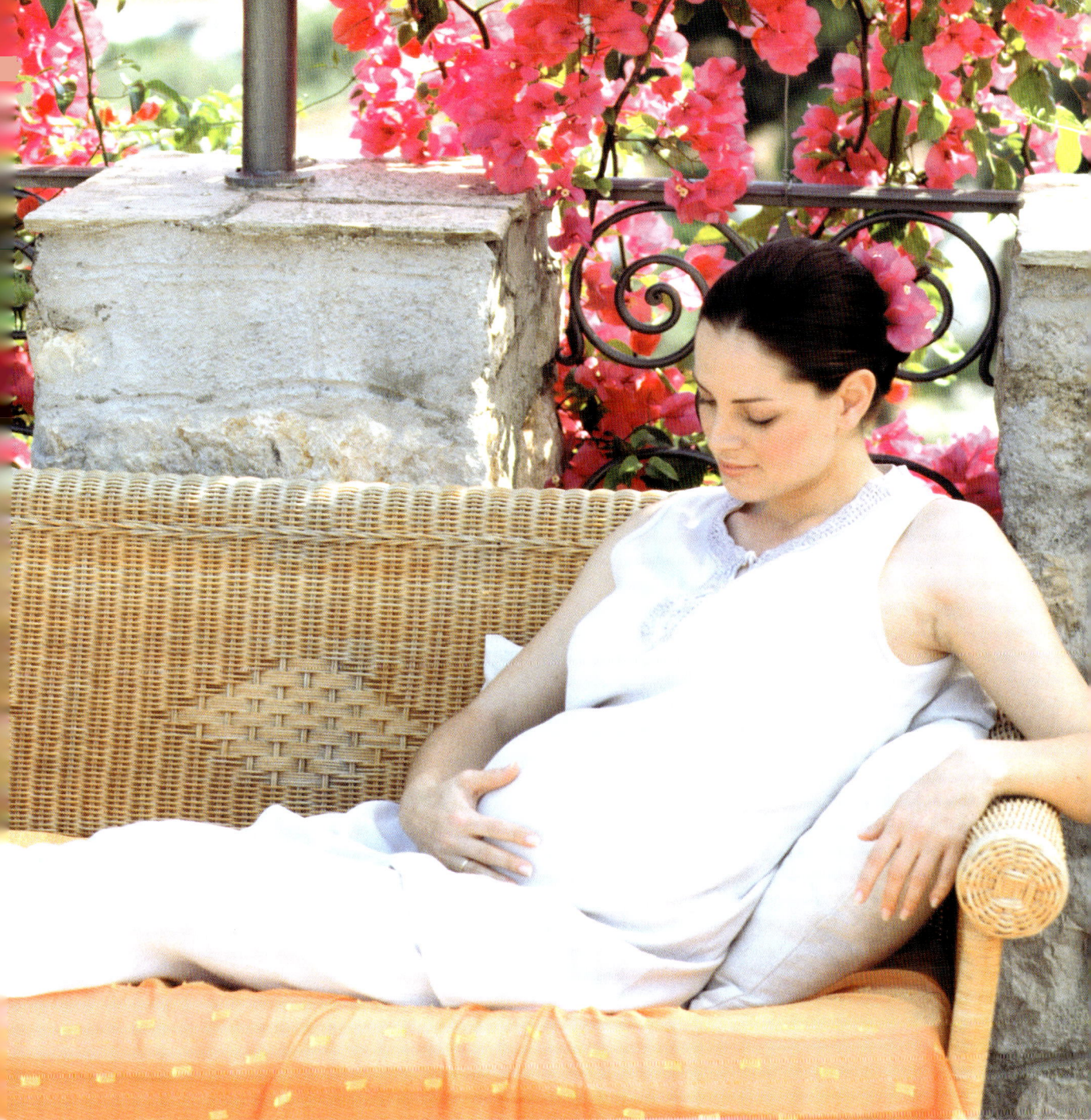

DISCLAIMER

Although the author and publishers have made every effort to ensure that the information contained in this book was accurate at the time of going to press, they accept no responsibility for any loss, injury or inconvenience sustained by any person using this book or following the advice given in it.

This book is dedicated to
The Unborn

CONTENTS

PREPARING FOR CHANGE   8

BREATHING AND RELAXATION   18

GUIDELINES FOR PRACTICE   28

SITTING AND SUPINE POSTURES   36

STANDING POSTURES   58

INVERTED POSTURES   70

POSTNATAL POSTURES   80

PLANNING YOUR OWN YOGA SESSIONS 92

CONTACTS AND INDEX   94

ACKNOWLEDGEMENTS AND CREDITS   96

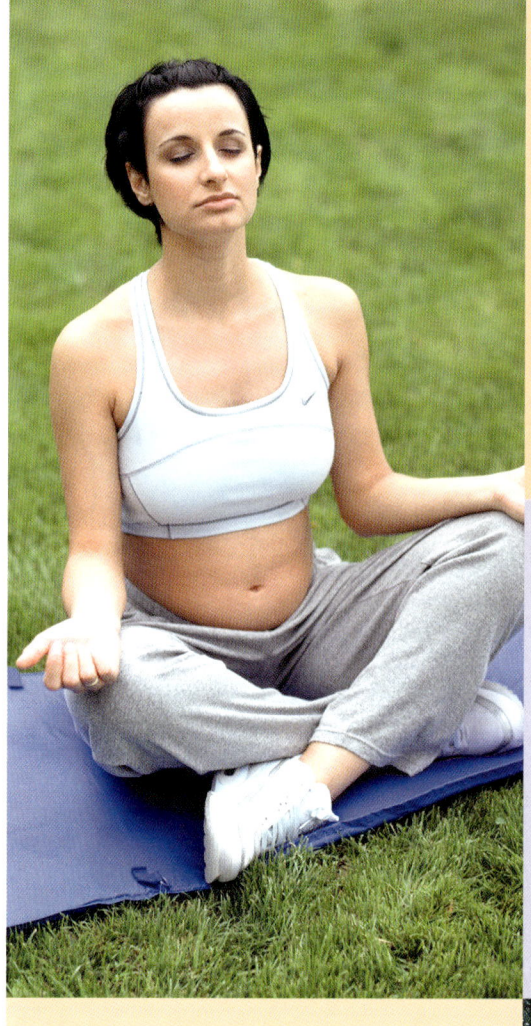

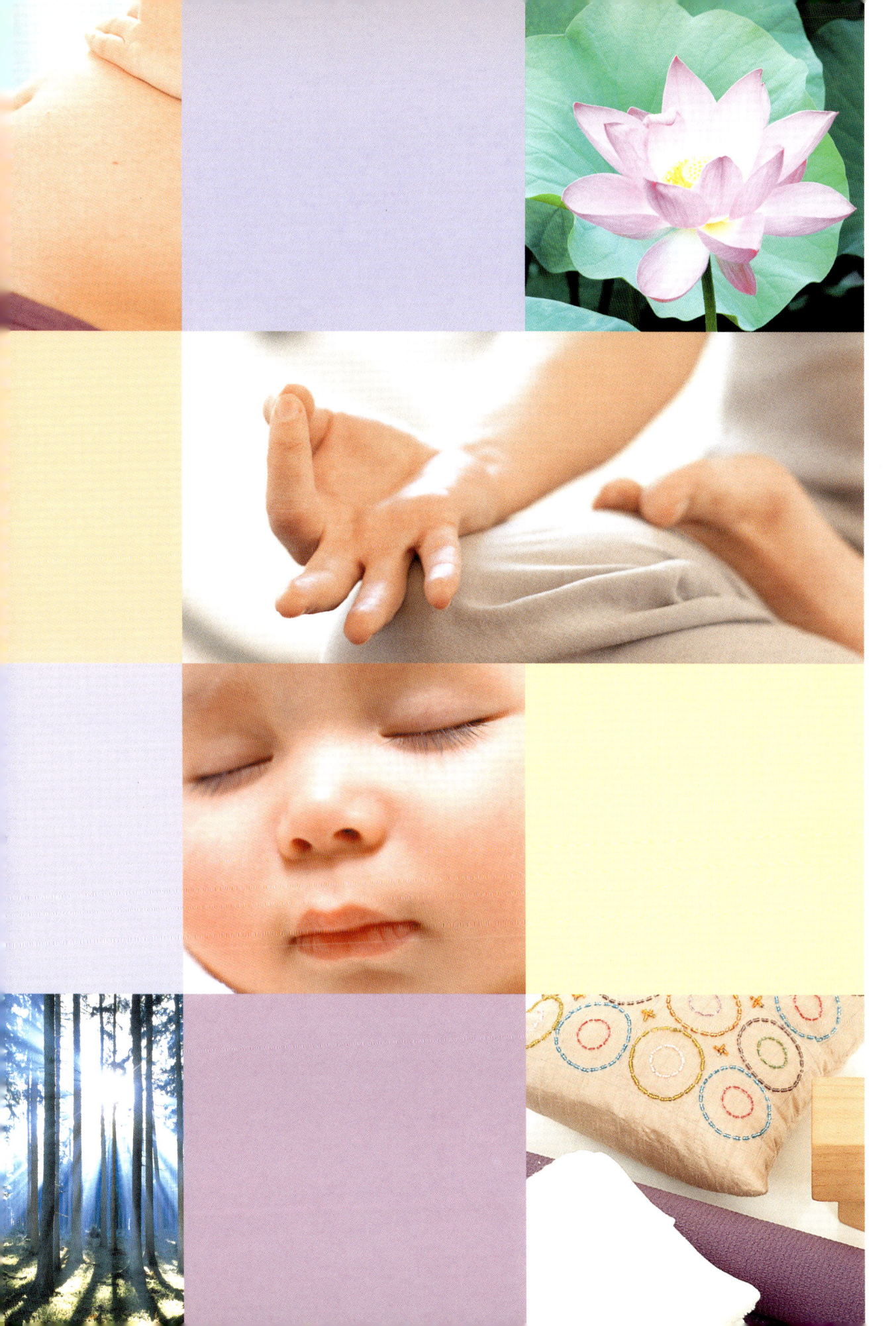

From conception until delivery, a pregnant woman's body and mind undergo a series of profound changes. Not only does she have to accommodate the growing foetus, but she has to adapt to the concept of motherhood and all it entails. Bringing a child into the world is possibly the most significant event in any woman's life. Giving birth is not just a passing thing, it is sure to affect you forever and your attitude to your pregnancy is vital.

From the time a foetus is fully formed it experiences all the mother's emotions. Although these emotions are not consciously registered by the baby, the hormones that produce joy or sorrow, sadness or happiness, wash over the foetus. Your emotional state is therefore of the utmost importance while you are carrying your child.

One of the functions of yoga is to bring about a balance between the body, mind and spirit. During your pregnancy you should aim to be as physically healthy and emotionally well-balanced as possible. Practising yoga will bring confidence, balance and harmony to your life and can have a dramatic effect on your overall wellbeing and attitude.

Preparing for Change

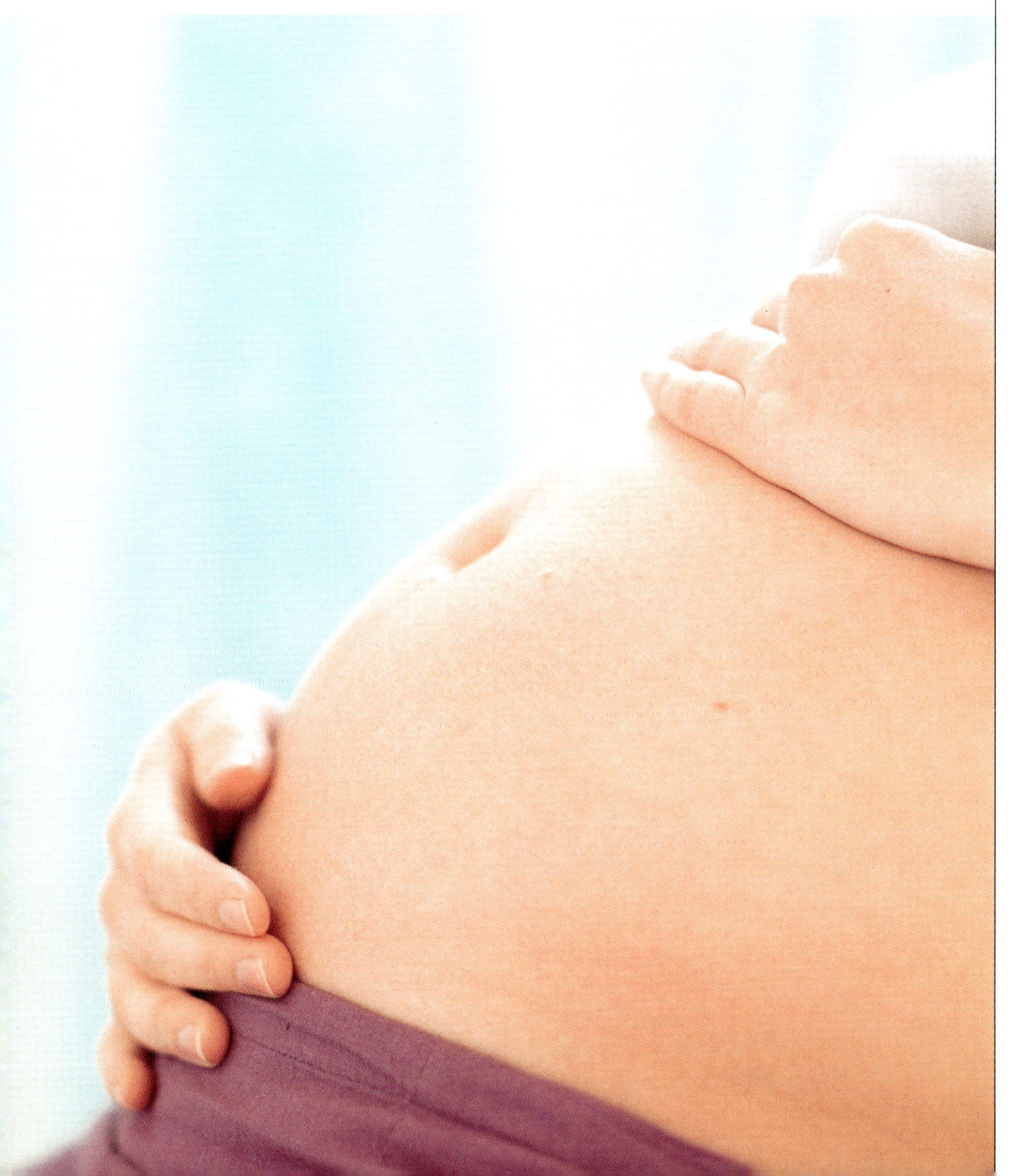

Preparing for Change

Yoga puts you intuitively in touch with your body, which is just what a pregnant woman needs. Professional advice is necessary during pregnancy and childbirth, but a woman's natural instincts and self-awareness are absolutely essential and yoga can assist in bringing about a calm confidence.

This practical guide is based on the principles of Hatha Yoga. The postures have been carefully chosen because they are absolutely safe for, and beneficial to, pregnant women. They will help to bring flexibility to the hips, pelvis and spine, as well as strengthen the entire body. The aim is to assist the future mother to be supple, strong, emotionally resilient and joyful.

Most of the exercises can be practised for the duration of pregnancy. Each posture is accompanied by a symbol indicating whether it is suitable for beginner, intermediate or advanced (B, I, A) students and whether it can be safely practised in the first, second or third trimester (1, 2, 3) or postnatally (P).

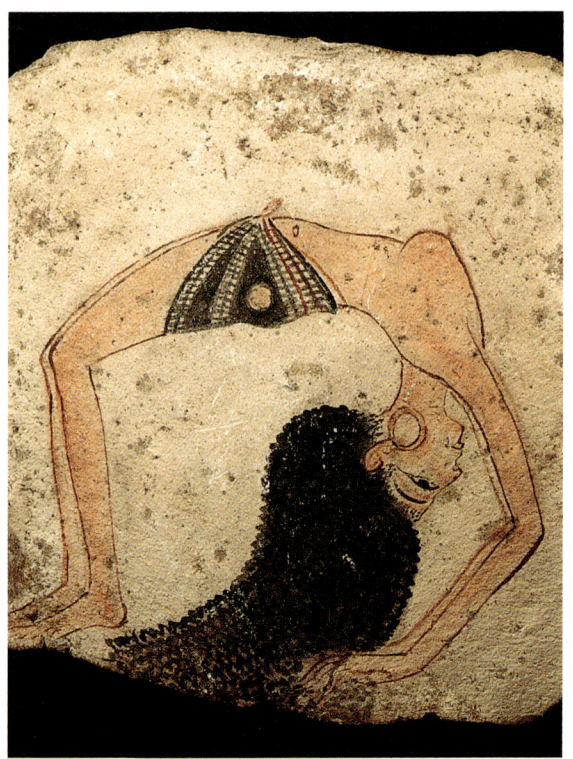

WHAT IS YOGA?

Yoga is a philosophical system, not a religion or faith. It has been practised in the East for more than 5000 years and is documented in the *Vedas*, the most sacred of the Hindu scriptures, which were written around 2000BC, and take the form of a series of hymns. Early evidence of yoga practice comes from carved stone seals, dating as far back as 3000BC, which demonstrate yoga postures.

Yoga is based on a combination of techniques which have a subtle effect on the entire person, influencing the body, the intellect and the emotions. In the West, yoga is most often practised as a system of mental and physical exercise, and induced relaxation which can be undertaken by anyone, regardless of their beliefs.

The word 'yoga' originated in Sanskrit as *joug* or *yuj*, which means 'yoke' or 'union'. In yogic thought this could be either man yoking himself to the Divine, or the joining, in a balanced manner, of all the different aspects which make up a human being. It has filtered through to English as the word 'conjugal', which relates to the mutual relationship between husband and wife.

There are five main paths, or branches, of yoga, which are interlinked yet separate. The first path is Raja Yoga, more commonly known as meditation. The next is Hatha Yoga, which is the practice of postures (asanas) and correct breathing (pranayama), both of which will be explored further in this book. Bhakti Yoga is the yoga of love and devotion, Jnana Yoga is the yoga of wisdom, and Karma Yoga is the yoga of cause and effect.

Top The 'om' sign (in shadow behind the text) represents the trinity of the three key Hindu gods, Brahma, Vishnu and Siva. It is a sacred sound that is used in meditation and prayer.
Left Yoga offers a bridge between mankind and the Divine, and has been practised since the earliest times.

The word 'hatha' is made up of two roots; 'ha' meaning 'sun' and 'tha' meaning 'moon'. The practice of Hatha Yoga is thus said to balance the solar and lunar energies within a person. Some people take it to mean balancing the male and female energies, the yin and yang. It can also refer to balancing positive and negative energies.

The ancient yoga texts set out certain rules, or guidelines, to be followed in the practice of yoga. If you examine them carefully it can be seen that they are the basic ethics of humanity and are probably followed by every society in the world. These moral rules or principles are divided into restraints, called yamas, and observances (niyamanas). The restraints are non-violence, honesty and truthfulness, moderation in all things, lack of possessiveness and not stealing. The observances are cleanliness, contentment, purity, austerity, selflessness, dedication and keeping company with learned and wise people.

CAUTION

Regardless of whether you have done yoga before, or are starting it for the first time, it is essential that you have the approval of your doctor or midwife, and are under the guidance of a qualified yoga teacher who is experienced in teaching yoga for pregnancy.

If you have been doing yoga for some time, or are a regular exerciser, it is possible to continue with a light routine during the first trimester. However, if you have never done yoga before, do not exercise, or have a history of miscarriage, you should not begin yoga exercises until the second trimester (after the 14th week of your pregnancy).

BENEFITS OF YOGA

Pregnant women are often discouraged from performing any strenuous physical exercise during the first trimester, particularly if there is any possibility of miscarriage, and are advised to commence an exercise programme only from the fourth month onwards. However, an active and healthy mother-to-be, who has no history of miscarriage, can start gently strengthening her body and developing suppleness and good muscle tone as soon as she feels ready.

You can practise yoga throughout your pregnancy by adapting the postures to suit your individual needs and level of fitness. These vary from person to person, so it is necessary to be in tune with your body, note any discomfort which may arise, and alter the positions to suit yourself.

For pregnant women, the physical benefits of yoga include improved strength, muscle tone, posture and balance; suppleness and flexibility in the entire muscular system; the stimulation of the glands which control hormone production; increased blood flow and improved circulation; and excellent breath control. During yoga practice, the internal organs are massaged. Furthermore, the stomach exercises (see pp82–84) will help you regain your figure after giving birth. Yoga helps to reduce sleeping problems and insomnia, and it promotes a general feeling of wellbeing and a positive outlook on life. Yoga also teaches self-observation, and practising it puts you intuitively in touch with your body and emotions.

Remember, though, yoga is not an exclusive recipe for a perfect pregnancy and birth. It is a tool that can help you during this exciting time and hopefully enhance the overall experience. The term 'labour' means hard work, and most women approach the labour of birth with some fear and trepidation. This is quite normal but, hopefully, yoga can make your pregnancy and labour a little easier and help you approach them with a feeling of calm control.

Preparing for Change

Your changing body

During pregnancy, the volume of blood circulating through a woman's body increases from approximately 5 litres (9 pints) to about 6.5 litres (11.5 pints) by the end of pregnancy. Although the pumping ability of the heart increases to cope with the greater volume of blood, the heart rate (the speed at which your heart beats) and blood pressure (the pressure the blood exerts on the walls of the arteries) should remain the same. As a result of the heart having to work harder, you may experience shortness of breath. The exercises in the chapter on yoga breathing (see p22), should help you to overcome this.

During pregnancy, specific hormones are produced which relax and widen the blood vessels. These hormones can also cause valves in the larger veins to soften, which can lead to varicose veins in the legs. Some yoga postures strengthen the heart and aid blood flow, as well as help prevent varicose veins. If veins do become enlarged, practising the Fountain posture, will help to reduce swelling.

Along with the increased amount of blood in the system comes an increase in the fluid content of the body's tissues and cells. During pregnancy, your body will retain up to 7 litres (12 pints) of excess water, amounting to approximately half of your total weight gain. Some of this excess fluid can collect in the feet and the ankles, causing them to swell, but this can also be relieved by practising the Fountain.

The pelvic ligaments and joints soften during pregnancy due to the action of the hormones progesterone and relaxin. This softening allows the body to become more flexible so that it can make space for the growing foetus. During labour, it also enables the ligaments which support the uterus to expand. Because your pelvic ligaments are softer, they need to be protected by strong, well-toned abdominal muscles. Yoga is an ideal way to tone and strengthen not only these muscles, but also the arteries that feed them.

The mother's frame has to carry the extra weight of a growing child, and this can put strain on the lower spine if the back muscles have not been strengthened. Her feet and legs also have to bear more weight and, once the child is born, she will carry an ever-increasing weight in her arms.

As the pregnancy advances, the uterus expands to accommodate the growing foetus. Furthermore, the muscles of the uterus are exceedingly active during the contractions of birth. There are specific exercises that strengthen the pelvic muscles and open the hip area to help support the uterus (see pp 40, 41, 43, 44).

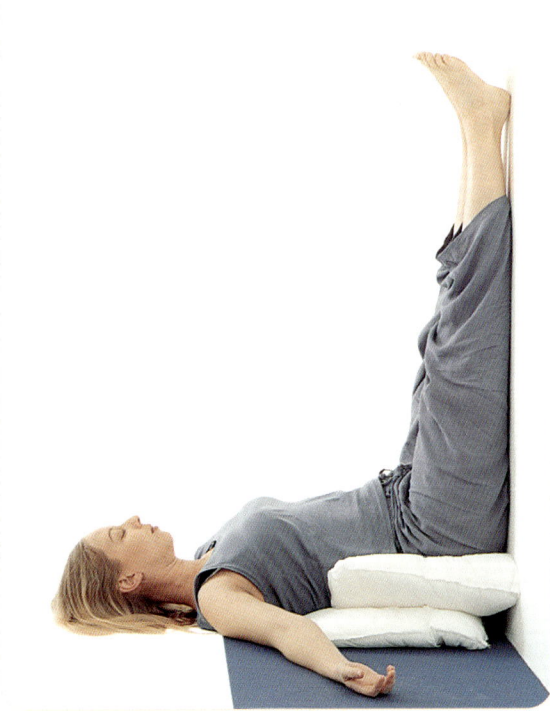

Above **The Fountain is a relaxing rest pose, particularly after a long day. It is especially beneficial for women who suffer from varicose veins or other leg problems.**

Your Changing Body

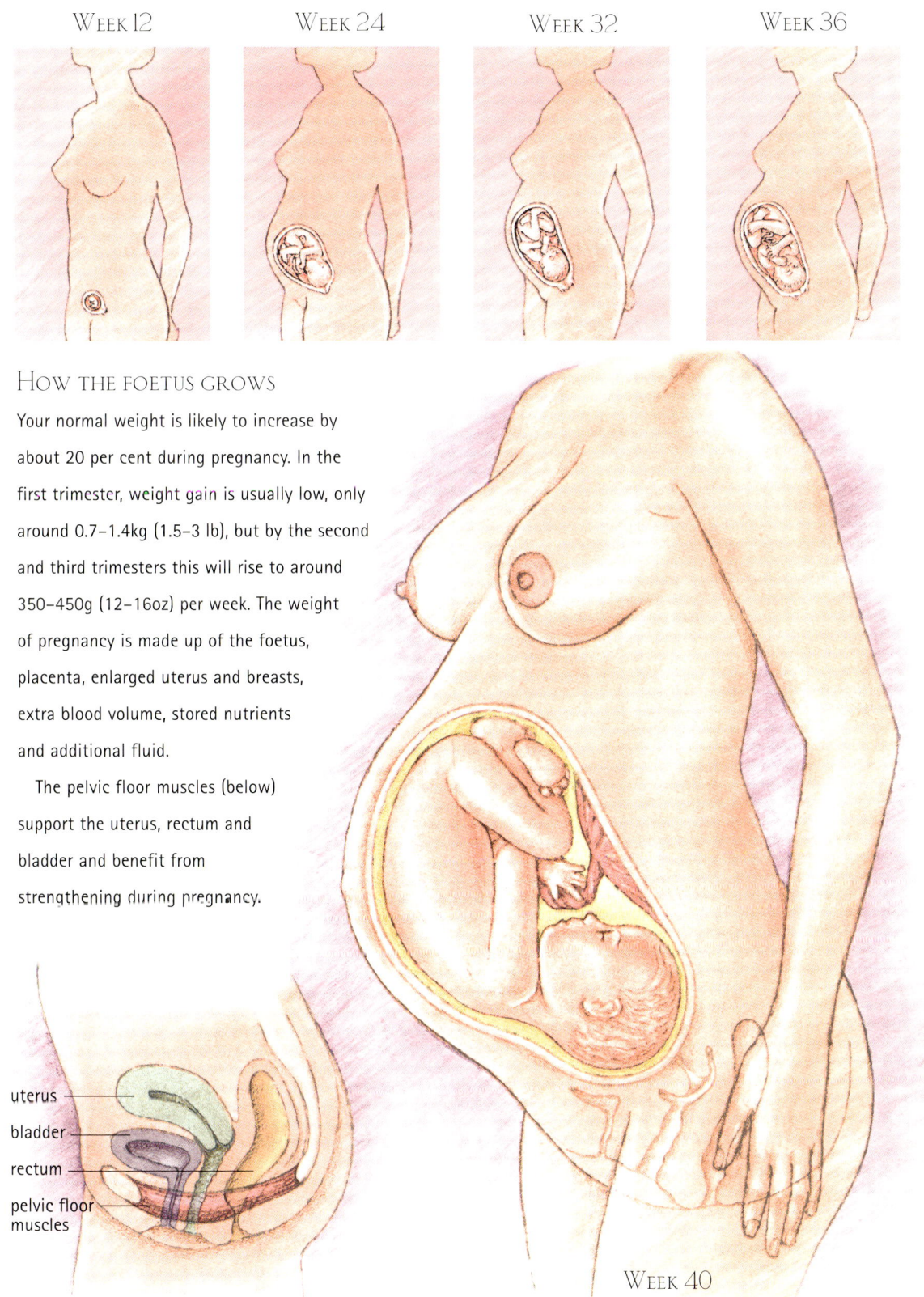

WEEK 12   WEEK 24   WEEK 32   WEEK 36

How the foetus grows

Your normal weight is likely to increase by about 20 per cent during pregnancy. In the first trimester, weight gain is usually low, only around 0.7–1.4kg (1.5–3 lb), but by the second and third trimesters this will rise to around 350–450g (12–16oz) per week. The weight of pregnancy is made up of the foetus, placenta, enlarged uterus and breasts, extra blood volume, stored nutrients and additional fluid.

The pelvic floor muscles (below) support the uterus, rectum and bladder and benefit from strengthening during pregnancy.

uterus
bladder
rectum
pelvic floor muscles

WEEK 40

Preparing for Change

Hormones and emotions

Many emotions are induced by chemical changes that take place in the brain. Throughout your pregnancy, you may find yourself more susceptible than usual to emotional upsets and unpredictable mood swings. This is due to the increased production of hormones, the body's chemical messengers. Hormones are produced by the endocrine glands (see illustration) and are transported around the body by the bloodstream. Hormones ensure the smooth functioning of your organs and, in women, are responsible for triggering the menstrual cycle, maintaining pregnancy and regulating labour, birth and breastfeeding.

The pituitary gland affects the functioning of the other endocrine glands and plays a role in the production of endorphins, the body's natural painkillers, which are essential during labour and have an all-round positive effect on your wellbeing. Postures such as the Headstand (see p78) and the Plough (see p76) stimulate the pituitary gland. (Neither posture should be practised during the last trimester.)

One of the hormones activated in pregnancy, prolactin, is secreted by the pituitary gland. Together with oestrogen and progesterone, prolactin is vital in stimulating the production of breast milk. Among other functions, oestrogen and progesterone relax the smooth muscle of the uterus, helping it to accommodate the growing foetus.

The production of adrenaline (epinephrine), noradrenaline (norepinephrine) and cortisone increases during pregnancy. Adrenaline and noradrenaline both alter the heart rate and blood pressure. Adrenaline also raises blood sugar levels by stimulating glucose production. Cortisone is a natural immunosuppressant which helps to relieve allergic reactions that occur during pregnancy. These hormones are produced by the adrenal glands, which are situated above the kidneys.

The load on the kidneys increases during pregnancy as they have to filter waste from both mother and foetus.

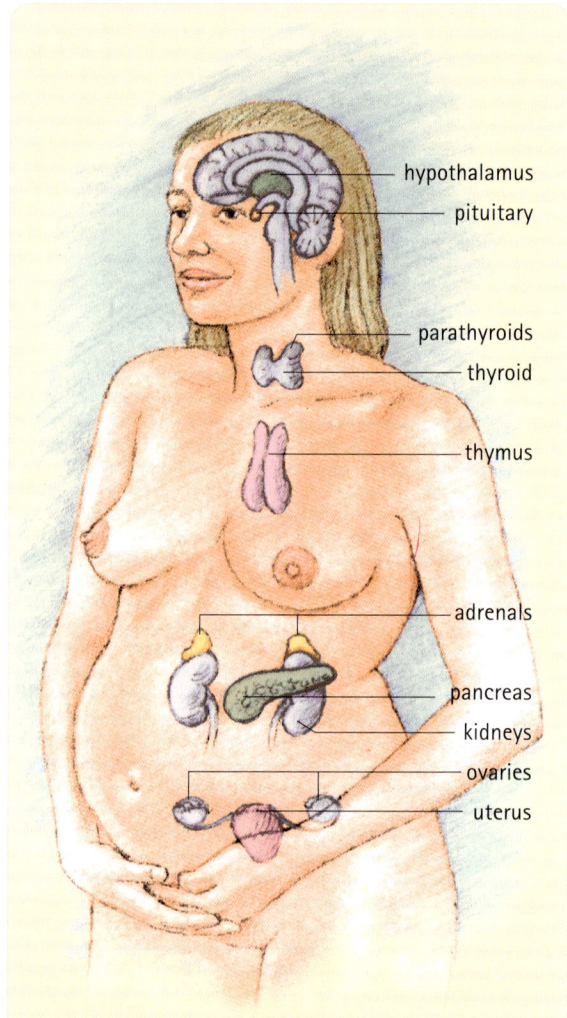

Endocrine system

The endocrine glands include the ovaries, thyroid, hypothalamus and adrenal glands. The pituitary gland, which is situated in the centre of the brain, is called the master endocrine gland as it affects the functioning of the other endocrine glands. Hormones produced by the endocrine glands ensure the smooth functioning of the body's organs.

Hormones and Emotions

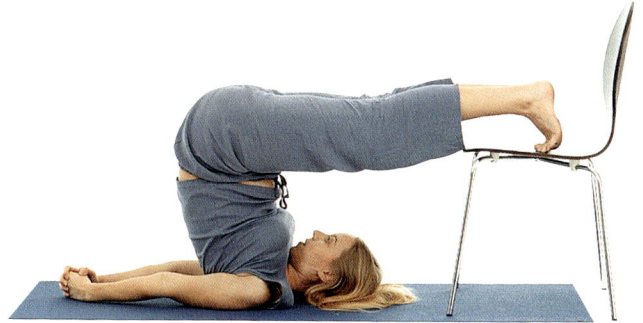
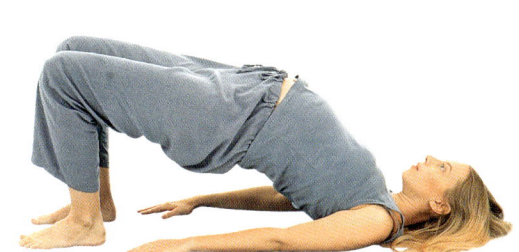

Above The Plough (p76), activates the pituitary gland – the master endocrine gland.
Above right Backbends, such as the Bridge (p48), help balance the production of hormones.

Gentle backbends (see p48) enable the kidneys to function better and also help to balance the production of hormones.

The hormone relaxin, which is produced by the placenta, causes the ligaments and connective tissues in the pelvis and uterus to become more elastic and flexible in preparation for birth. You should not over-stretch these ligaments though, so avoid extreme twists or backbends.

Breath control is an important part of yoga. Apart from being able to function more efficiently, if you can control your breathing, you will find it easier to manage your body and emotions. When you get angry or upset, adrenaline flows and your heart rate and blood pressure increase. As you lose control of your emotions, you may cry or say things you later regret. If, at the beginning of a conflict you consciously take control of your breath, you will find it easier to manage your body and emotions.

Practising yoga will improve your wellbeing and promote calmness, while learning to breathe correctly (see p21) will help you during labour.

CHAKRAS

Energy centres, or chakras, are situated throughout the body. Energy (prana) flows along channels (nadis), which intersect at the chakras. Each chakra is associated with a colour, organ, endocrine gland, and physical or emotional functions, as outlined below.

- **Crown** Purple. Brain. Pineal gland. Faith, enlightenment and higher consciousness.
- **Brow** Indigo. Brain. Pituitary and hypothalamus. Wisdom and awareness of the mind.
- **Throat** Blue. Metabolism. Thyroid and parathyroid. Communication with others and within oneself.
- **Heart** Green. Heart and lungs. Thymus. Cardiovascular (circulation and respiration), compassion and passion.
- **Solar plexus** Yellow. Pancreas, stomach and liver. Emotions and self-awareness.
- **Navel** Orange. Kidneys and intestines. Adrenal glands. Digestion and nourishment.
- **Base** Red. Gonads. Reproductive organs. Source of energy.

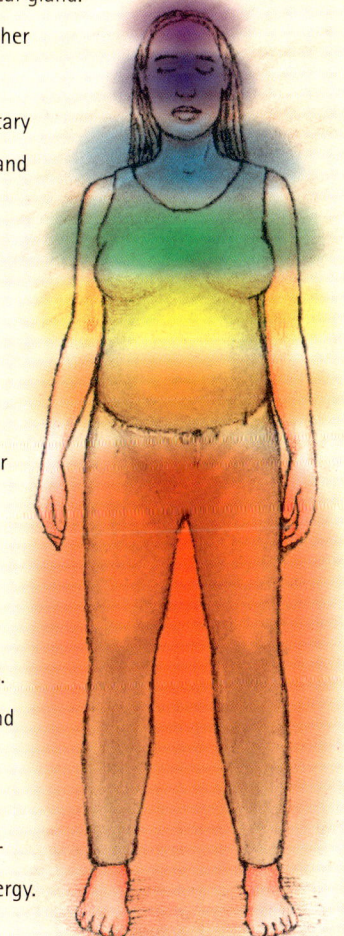

Preparing for Change

Preparing for labour

Labour is not something you can practise and, in any case, every labour is different. A long labour might be easy, while a short labour could be difficult. Practising yoga during your pregnancy will help you gain control over your body, which you otherwise would not have had. It is not easy to relax your muscles when you are in pain and it is often difficult to breathe when your body is under stress, but yoga will help you instinctively to let go and relax when you should, and to work with your body and gravity when you must bear down.

Your emotional preparations for labour are important and yoga can assist by promoting a positive attitude and helping to lessen the fear of pain. However, no matter how much you anticipate and plan for labour, when your time comes, it is best to tune into your body and do what feels most natural.

As your delivery date approaches, you should keep yourself busy. Sitting around waiting for the big day can lead to tension and stress, particularly if the baby does not arrive on the due date. It is important though, to get sufficient rest in the final weeks.

The first phase of labour begins with contractions, which continue and increase in intensity until the cervix dilates. This is usually the longest phase. The second phase occurs when the cervix is fully dilated and the baby's head begins to appear, followed by the body. The third phase is the loosening and expulsion of the placenta. Now the real bonding between mother and child can begin.

When your contractions begin, take a warm bath, or listen to some gentle music to get you into a relaxed mood, so that by the time the more intense contractions occur you are already in tune with the internal rhythms of your body. (Some women even doze between contractions in the first stages of labour.) You should also move around as much as possible, adopting positions that ease your contractions, either on your own or with the support of your birth partner. Towards the end of labour your body will simply take over and do what is required of it in the most amazing way. This is when you can really experience your body at its most creative, the way women have been doing for centuries.

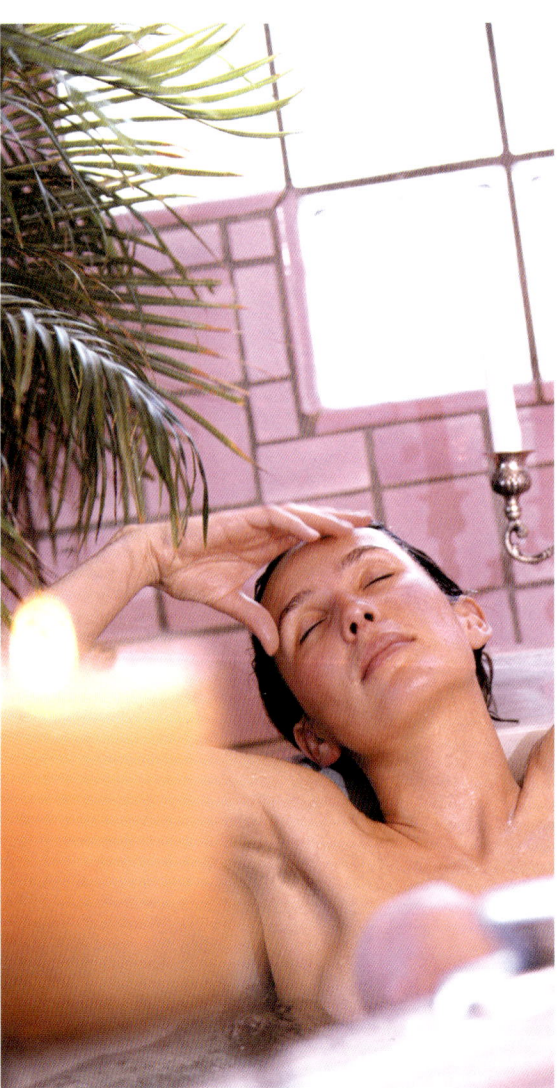

Left **A warm bath can have a wonderfully soothing effect in the early stages of labour, allowing you to relax momentarily before the hard work of the final phase begins.**

Preparing for Labour

Postures for labour

Many doctors prefer a woman to give birth while lying on her back, as this position makes things easier for the doctor, but labour is often easiest for the mother if she has gravity working for her. In other words, the vagina should be facing down towards the earth. Lying on the back places pressure on the large nerves in the spine, causing much of the pain involved in labour, and on the blood vessels which supply the uterus and the placenta, thus diminishing the blood flow.

One of the most natural positions in which to give birth is a supported squat (see p35), but kneeling on all fours, as in the Cat Stretch posture (see p46), is another option. In early labour, the Cobbler's Pose (see p42), or just sitting cross-legged, can be very comfortable. Right up to the final stages of labour, it is important to be able to move around.

Breathing during labour

Breathing helps to control pain and breathing correctly will benefit you enormously during labour. In the first phase, when your contractions start, find a position that is naturally comfortable and focus your awareness on your breathing. Concentrate on exhaling, imagining that you are breathing out all your tension and pain.

When a contraction begins, take in a long, slow breath, then exhale as slowly as possible, until the contraction is over. The contraction will be like a wave reaching its peak and then ebbing away. Do not try to anticipate the next contraction. Keep your mind focused on what is happening at the present time and try to go with it.

Making a noise during labour can be beneficial as it will also help to ease any pain. Do not feel inhibited. When your jaw opens for a sound to come out, your vagina will relax, but clenching your teeth will have the effect of tightening the cervical muscles. Gentle rhythmical swaying from side to side, or rocking backwards and forwards, also helps to relax the abdominal muscles and reduce pain. Throughout labour, ensure that your body is always in the most comfortable position possible. Lie down, and play the same music you normally listen to while relaxing after a yoga session, as your brain is conditioned to relax under these conditions.

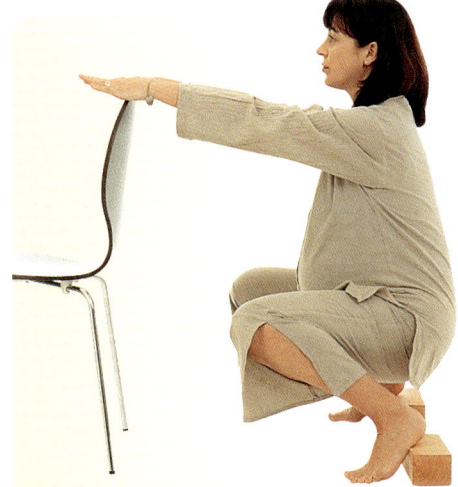

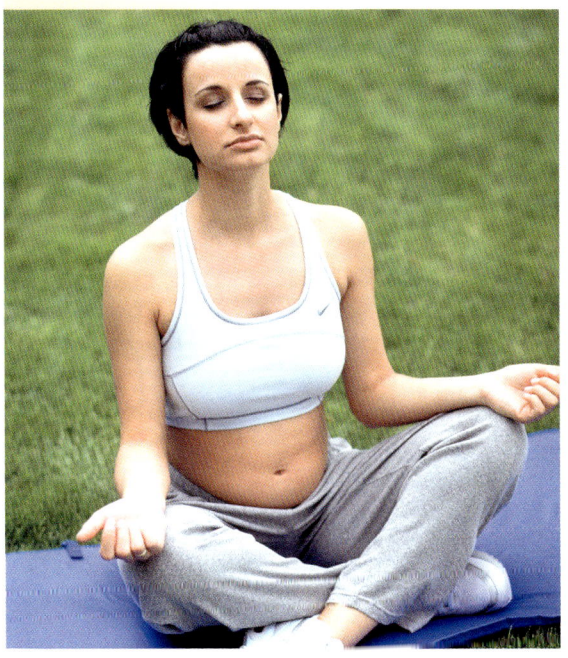

Above **Breathing is a key to controlling pain during labour. Regular practice beforehand will pay dividends on the day.**
Top **Many women choose to give birth in a squatting position, as it enables them to use the force of gravity.**

17

WHEN we breathe air, absorb sunlight, eat food, or drink water we absorb energy from these substances. In yoga, this vital energy, or life force, that keeps us functioning is called prana. The Chinese call it chi. Prana is in the air that we inhale, but it is not the oxygen; it is in the food we eat, but it is not the food itself. It is the subtle energy found in all things that keeps us alive.

An excellent way of explaining prana is to compare it to electricity. When you turn a light on, it shines, proving that energy is present, although you cannot see it. Everything and everyone exerts electromagnetic currents. Prana is the energy in our electromagnetic current. Through full active breathing and the practice of yoga postures, the body absorbs and stores more prana than usual which is what leaves you feeling so alive after a yoga session.

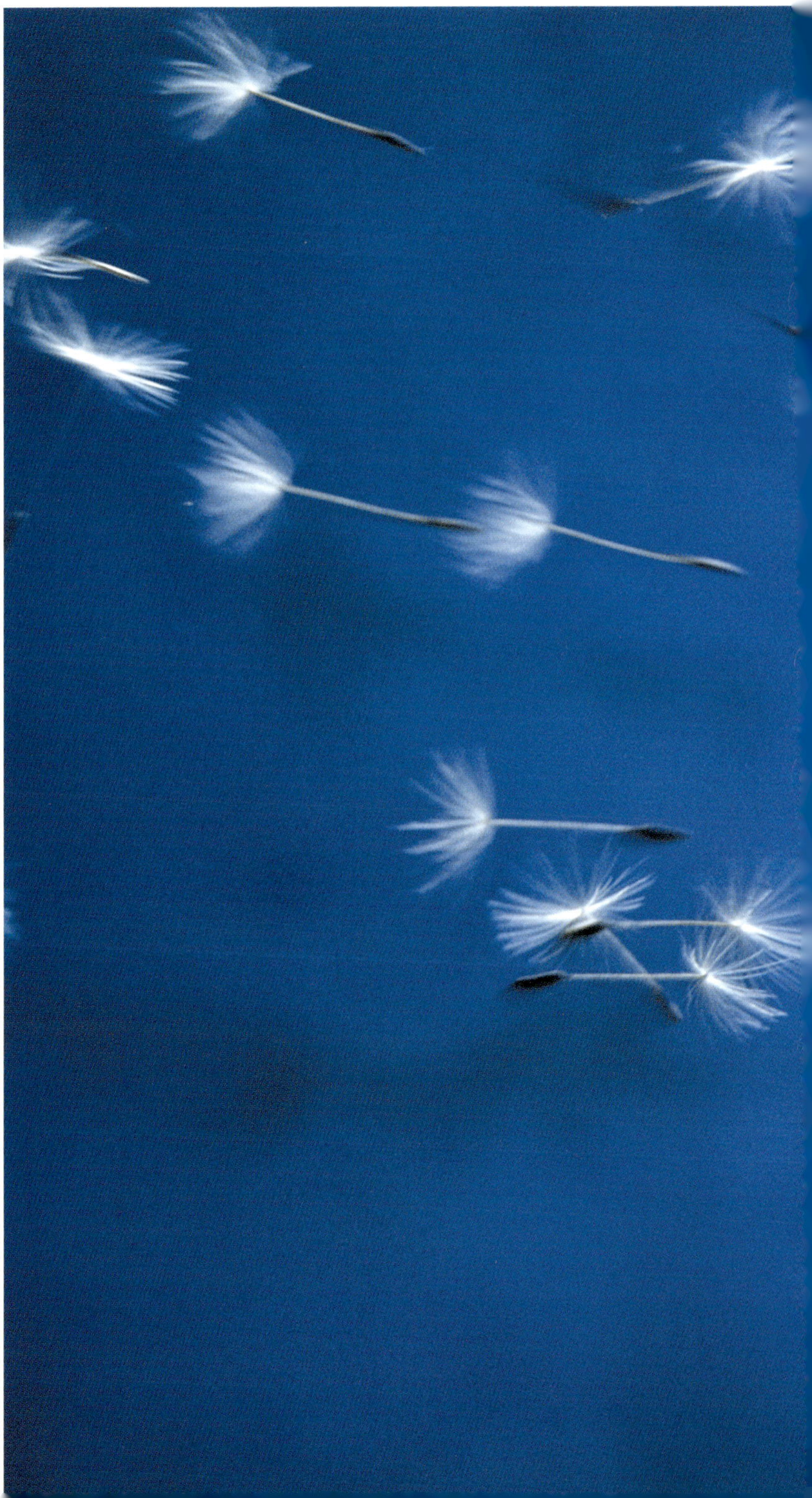

Breathing and Relaxation

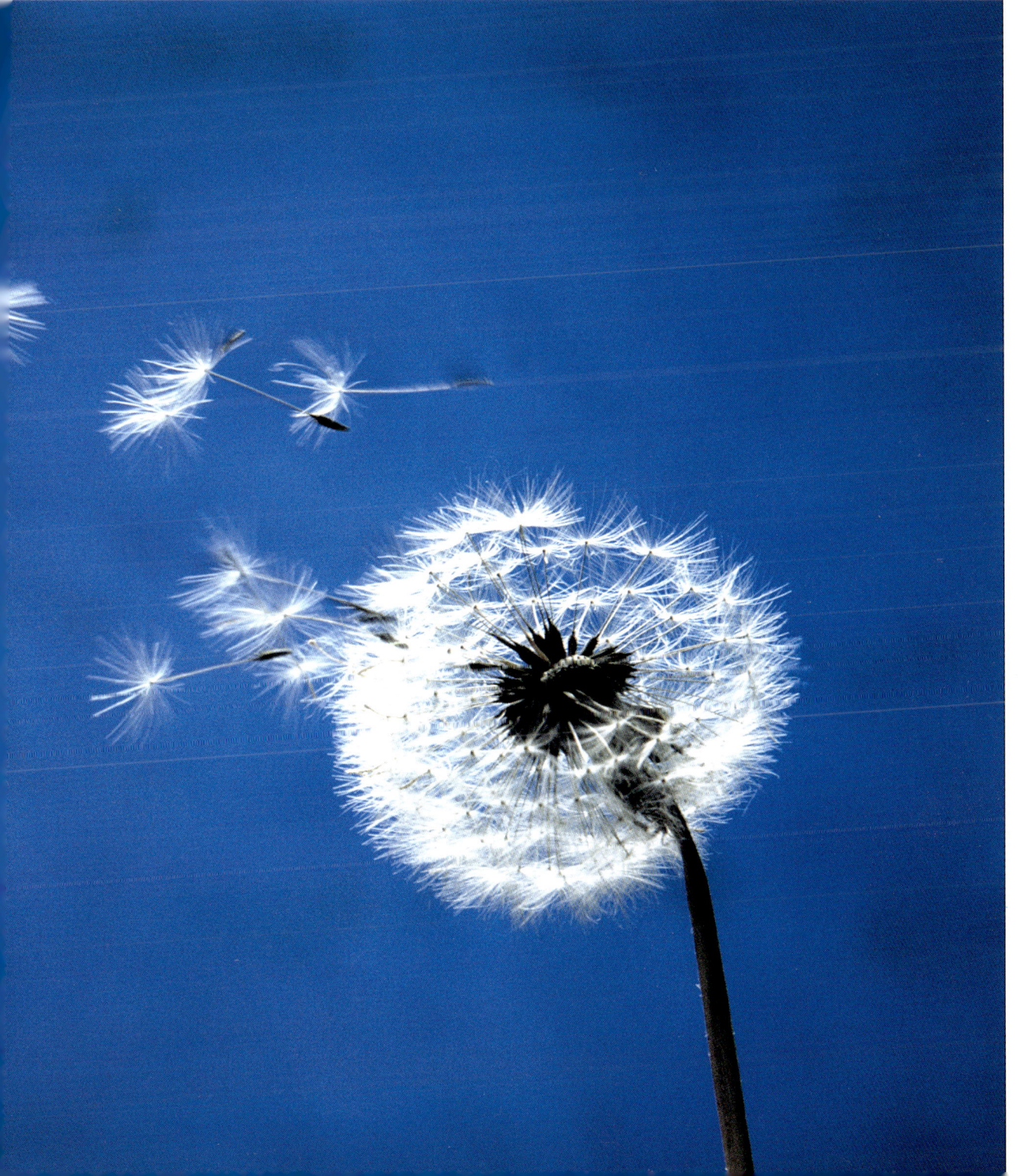

Breathing and Relaxation

Breathing keeps us alive. When the breath stops, life ceases to exist. When we inhale and absorb the correct amount of oxygen into our system, we function at peak performance.

The lungs take up almost the entire chest cavity, extending from underneath the collarbones to below the ribcage, where the diaphragm is situated, and through to the back, where the ribs attach to the spine.

When you inhale, you should fill your lungs from the bottom right up to the collarbones and all the way through to the back ribs. However, even under normal conditions, most people are habitually lazy breathers. If you watch your breathing carefully, you will probably find that you are breathing in only one area of the lungs.

Most lazy breathing is caused by bad habits, as well as by stress and tension. As soon as we are stressed, we tend to hold our breath, or breathe more shallowly, and our lungs act as if they want to go on strike. This means that the vitality of every cell in the body is diminished

The oxygen we breathe and the food we eat are converted into energy within the body. As this conversion takes place, toxins are formed which must be eliminated. Toxins are referred to as 'apana' and a posture called Apanasana (see p39) aids in the elimination process.

CAUTION

At various stages of your pregnancy you may experience a drop in blood pressure, shortness of breath, and feelings of lightheadedness or fainting, so take care when doing any breathing exercises.

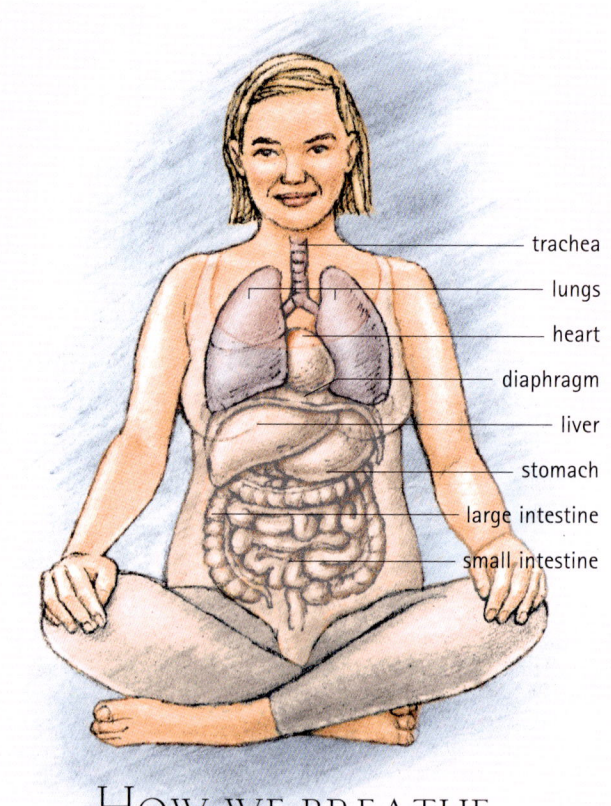

HOW WE BREATHE

When we inhale, oxygen passes through the windpipe into the lungs, which are made up of tiny air sacs, the alveoli, that are covered with a web of blood vessels. The oxygen passes from the alveoli into the blood vessels, from where it is transported by the red blood cells to every part of the body. Waste, in the form of carbon dioxide (CO_2), moves in the opposite direction and is eliminated as you exhale. A foetus is supplied with oxygen in exactly the same way, with the blood passing through the placenta. The mother exhales the baby's carbon dioxide along with her own breath.

The lungs expand on inhalation and contract on exhalation. The diaphragm, a muscle situated just below the ribcage, moves up and down with each exhalation and inhalation, respectively. As the diaphragm pushes down, it massages the liver, spleen and intestines, stimulating circulation throughout the entire abdominal area as well as to your baby.

Yoga breathing

In yoga, the practice of different breathing exercises is called Pranayama. Before attempting any form of yoga breathing, the first step is to learn how to breathe correctly.

CAUTION

There are many types of breathing exercises in yoga. Those given here are all safe to practise while you are pregnant. However, you should never hold your breath during pregnancy as the foetus requires oxygen at all times. If you are an experienced yoga practitioner, remember not to hold your breath, even for a short time, during any of the postures.

Correct breathing

Lie flat on a yoga mat or towel with your knees bent and touching each other and your feet wider apart than your hips. As your pregnancy advances, place a cushion or bolster under your knees for added comfort (1). When you are learning to breathe properly, lying down allows the body to relax. Bending the knees ensures that the diaphragm is in a relaxed position and allowing them to touch releases any stress from the small of the back. If your chin points towards the ceiling, causing the neck vertebrae to contract, place a cushion under your head. Make sure your teeth are not clenched and your tongue is soft in the base of your mouth, not stuck to the palate. It is difficult to relax when you are cold, so cover yourself with a blanket if necessary. (After 30 weeks, do this exercise sitting with your legs crossed.)

At first, don't do anything except observe the quality of your breath, watching to see if it is smooth, regular and even. Do not alter your breath, just observe it. Check to see which part of your lungs the air is flowing into.

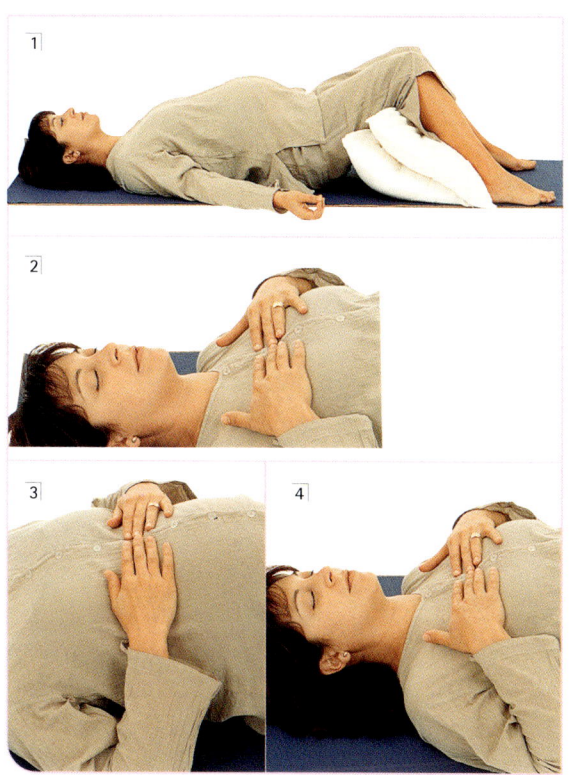

Place your hands lightly over your abdomen (2), inhale through your nose and consciously take the air to the area underneath your hands, allowing them to gently move away from each other. This is not an arm movement – let the breath move the hands. Take 10 long, controlled breaths, inhaling and exhaling through your nose. Move your hands higher, so that the middle fingers are touching each other just below your breasts (3). Take another 10 breaths, again consciously guiding the air to below your hands. There should be no stress in your arms, hands or shoulders. Now, move your hands to the area above your breasts but below your collarbones (4) and repeat the 10 breaths. Make a mental note of how it feels as the air flows into each part of your lungs. Allow your body to resume its natural breathing rhythm for 10 breaths and just relax. Place your arms alongside your body with the palms facing upwards.

Breathing and Relaxation

Next, take in a long, slow, controlled breath, filling first the bottom, then the middle and then the top of your lungs. Exhale, emptying the top of the lungs first, then the middle and then the bottom. Repeat this 10 times and then again allow your body to take on its natural breathing rhythm.

When doing this exercise, do not tense your shoulders, arms or jaw. Watch out for this, as tension creeps in when we are not observing it. Do not take in too much air in one breath because your shoulders will pull up and tense. There should be no stress at the edges of your breath (that is, at the end of the inhalation and exhalation). Try to make the switch from breathing in to breathing out as smooth as possible; the exercise should be calm and effortless. Always ensure that you exhale for a little longer than you inhale to avoid hyperventilation (getting dizzy or light-headed).

Breathing like this may feel a little weird when you first start to practise it, but bear in mind that breathing is as vital to the foetus as to the mother. With practice, regular correct breathing will become second nature, and it will stand you in good stead for the rest of your life. Breath control will be your biggest aid while giving birth. Once correct breathing becomes easy and comfortable, practise it while driving, watching TV or standing in the supermarket queue. If you don't have time for a full yoga session during the course of a day, at least practise correct breathing. This is an excellent exercise to practise with your partner.

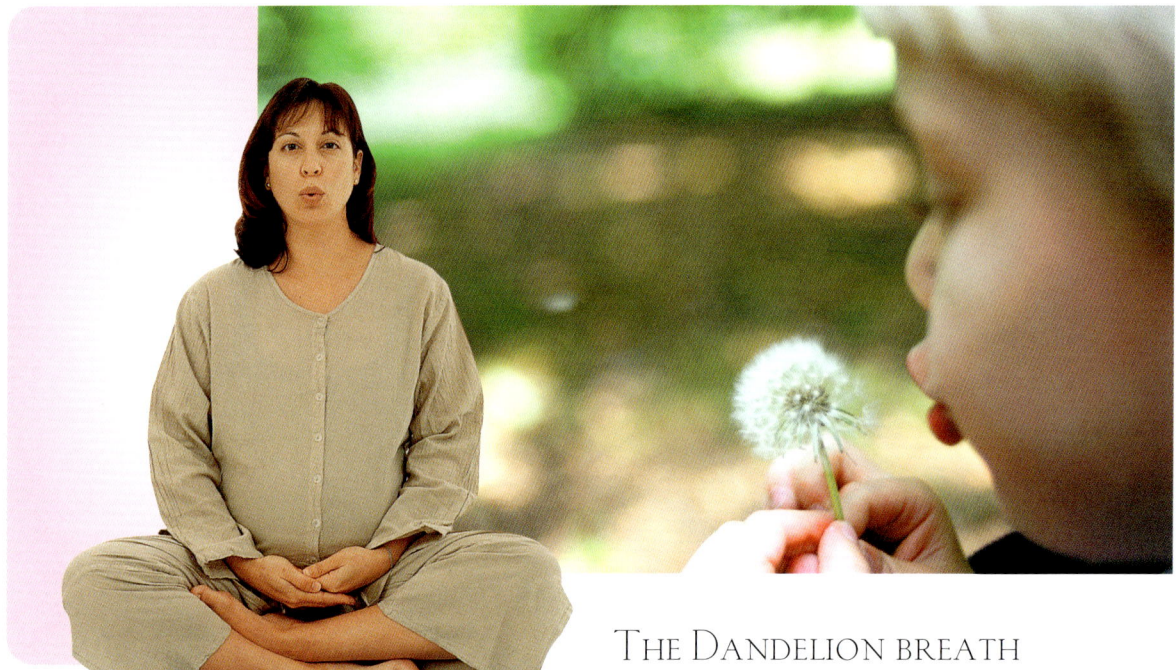

THE DANDELION BREATH

This breathing technique will help you in the first stages of labour. It is a gentle exercise that enhances breath control by helping you breathe out in a gentle manner. Think of a dandelion flower, with its soft fluffy calyx, or 'puff'. Children love blowing the seeds away and the same technique is used for this exercise. Sit in a comfortable position with your hands in your lap. Purse your lips and blow a little air out of your mouth as though you were blowing the dandelion seeds away. Continue exhaling with short, sharp breaths through your mouth until all the air is expelled. Inhale through your nose and repeat 15 times before taking a couple of recovery breaths. Repeat the entire exercise six times.

Brahmari (the humming bee)

Sit in the same position as for the previous exercise. Inhale through both nostrils and exhale through your nose. Hum loudly on the exhalation, keeping your mouth closed. Keep the exhalation and the humming going for as long as it remains comfortable, then inhale through your nose without humming. Repeat 10 times. Humming enables you to extend the exhalation period and enhances breath control.

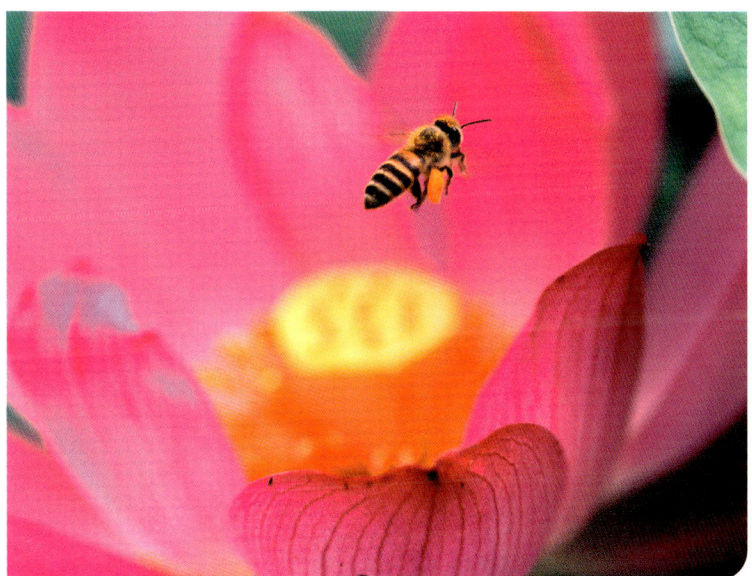

The humming also vibrates deep into the lung tissue, loosening congestion, so this is an excellent exercise for relieving any tightness in your chest. The Brahmari breath is exceptionally soothing and calming. Because of the extended exhalation, it is very beneficial to pregnant women and is a wonderful preparation for labour.

Ujjayi breathing (the yoga breath)

Ujjayi breathing is used in almost all yoga postures. This form of breathing can feel a little strange at first, but persevere, as it is the basis of all Hatha Yoga postures and allows one to move and breathe slowly and with control.

The easiest way to learn this breathing technique is to lie in the position for the correct breathing exercise (p21). All inhalation and exhalation is done through the nose and the mouth is kept closed.

The main characteristic of Ujjayi breathing is the partial closing of the windpipe with the glottis, which is located in the back of the throat. You do this by contracting the muscles at the base of your throat, near the collarbones.

Closing the glottis acts as a brake on the inflow and outflow of air, giving you greater control over the breath. Keeping the glottis contracted, draw the breath slowly down into the back of the throat and into the lungs.

As you inhale, fill the lungs from the bottom, moving to underneath the breasts and then up to the collarbones. A good analogy for this is filling a bottle with water: the bottom of the bottle fills first, then the middle and then finally the top. The air going down the back of the throat should create a slight sibilant (hissing) sound.

Exhale slowly through your nose, keeping the glottis partially closed. At all times during this exercise, your focus should be on the back of the throat, not in the nostrils. If you experience difficulty getting the hang of it, then sigh the air out of your mouth as though you were trying to mist a window pane, and notice the feeling of air in the back of your throat. Now practise doing this with your lips closed, but maintaining the focus of the breath in the throat, as opposed to in the nose. (Remember to exhale for slightly longer than you inhale, to avoid retaining too much oxygen, which might make you light-headed.)

Repeat the Ujjayi breath 10 times and then allow the body to resume its natural breathing rhythm for a while before doing another 10 rounds.

Breathing and Relaxation

Nadi Sodhana
(alternate nostril breathing)

One nostril is always more dominant than the other, with the air flowing more freely through it. This is normal and, in a healthy person, should change from the left nostril to the right and back again every two hours on average.

Sit in a comfortable position with your hands resting lightly in your lap (1). With your right hand, feel for the end of the septum (the soft part of your nose), as this is what you will be closing.

Fold the index and middle fingers of your right hand into the palm (2). Place your right thumb lightly against the septum on the right side of your nose to close the right nostril (3) and inhale gently through the left nostril. Then close the left nostril with the ring finger of the right hand, lift the thumb, and exhale through the right nostril (4). It is not necessary to apply pressure to the nose, a light touch is all that is required.

Keeping the left nostril closed, inhale through the right nostril. Close the right nostril with the thumb and exhale through the left nostril. Always start and end this exercise by inhaling and exhaling through the left nostril. The rhythm is always left, right, right, left. This comprises one round of Nadi Sodhana. Keep the right elbow lifted away from your ribcage throughout and the shoulders soft and free of tension.

Do 12 rounds of alternate nostril breathing and then relax for a while with your eyes closed to allow your body to resume its natural breathing rhythm. Nadi Sodhana is probably the most calming of all the yoga breathing exercises. It brings about a balance between the right and left hemispheres of the brain, inducing a wonderful feeling of serenity.

Nadi Sodhana is usually practised with breath retention, but as this is not recommended during pregnancy, keep your breathing steady throughout.

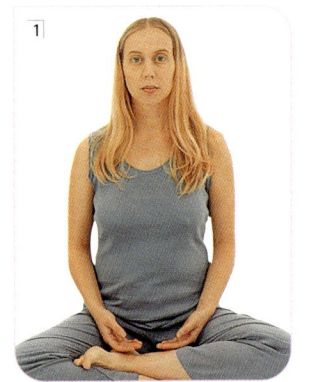
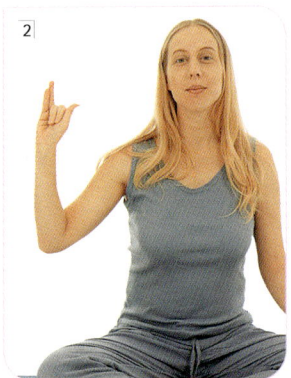
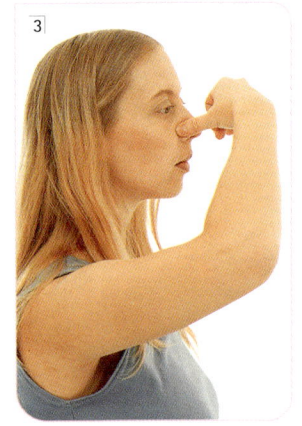
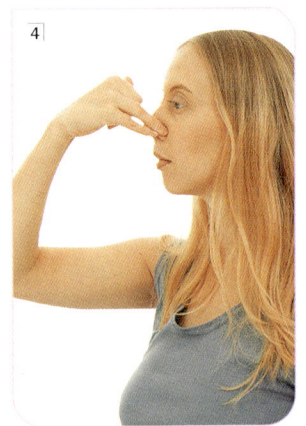
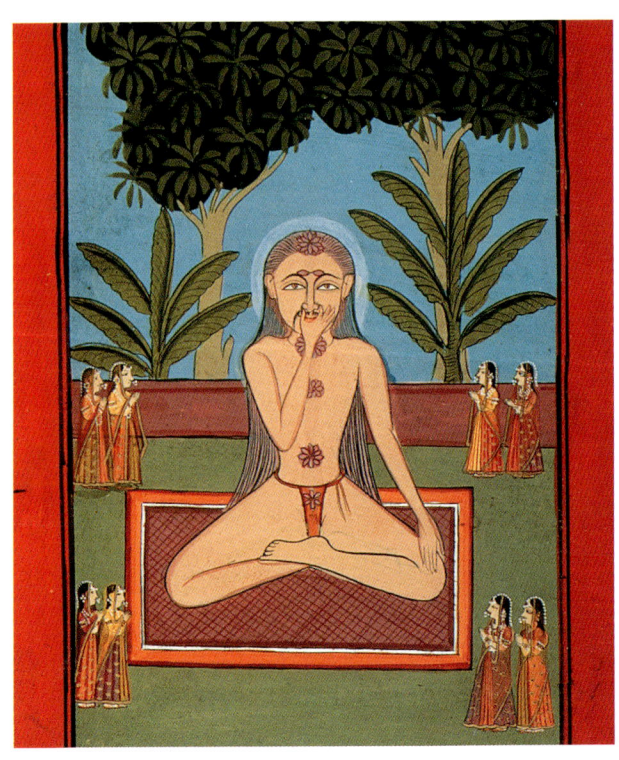

Chanting

Many people are put off by the idea of chanting as it makes them feel self-conscious. Have a look at the word 'self-conscious'. It can easily be replaced with 'self-awareness', which is one of the basic aims of yoga. Once you understand what chanting does and how it works on the body, maybe this reluctance can be overcome. Also remember that not everybody who practises yoga does chanting.

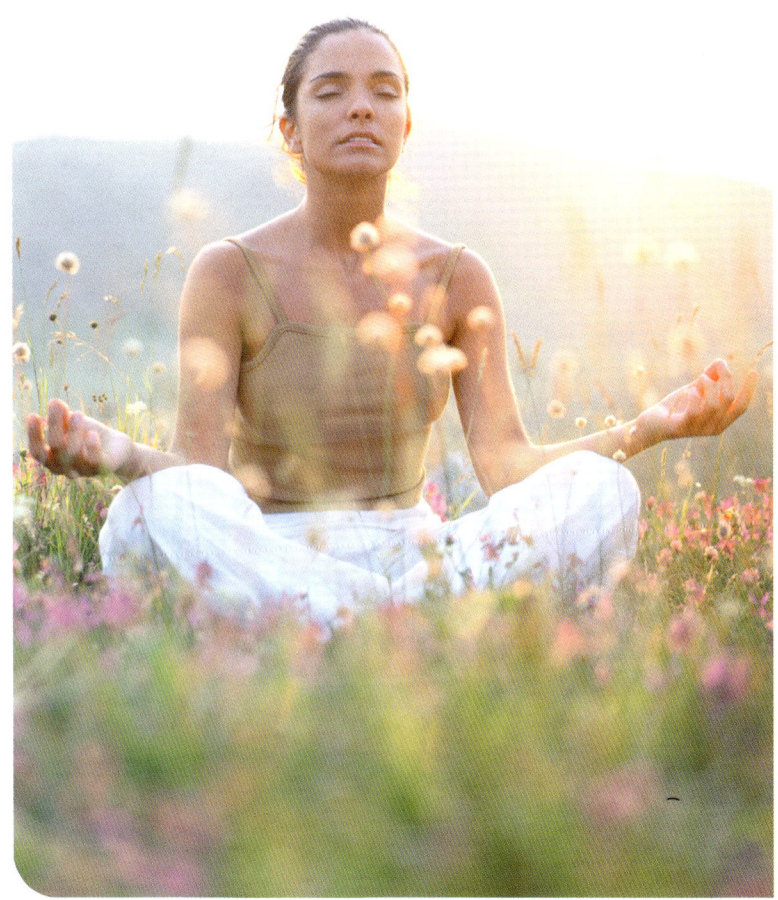

When you chant, you are setting up a vibration that reverberates through the whole upper body. Chanting stimulates the alveoli (air sacs) in the lungs, improving the exchange of gases (oxygen and carbon dioxide). It massages the internal organs, reaches into the deep-lying tissues and nerve cells, and enhances blood circulation.

The sound rises through the body from the base of the spine to the crown of the head. Along the way it stimulates the endocrine system, particularly the pineal and pituitary glands, which produce the chemicals that make us feel good (see p14).

If you want to try chanting, sit in a comfortable position with your hands resting lightly in your lap. Start with a simple chant, such as repeating the word Om, which Yogis consider to be the sound of creation.

Close your eyes and inhale through the nose. Open your mouth wide and breathing out through your mouth, slowly chant 'Om' (also written as Aum), splitting the word into three distinct sounds: aaahhh, ooohhh, and finally, mmmm, which is done with your mouth closed.

As the sound progresses you should be able to feel the vibration rising through your body. (You may not be able to feel it immediately, but with a little practice it will come.) To enhance the rising effect, draw your stomach muscles towards your spine on the 'ah' and the 'ooh', to force the sound up into the lungs. As the muscles are drawn further in, the sound will rise until it reaches the skull for the 'mm'. The 'mm' sound can be moved around the cranium by moving the jaw slowly, either up and down, or in a circle. If you place your hand on the crown of your head you will be able to feel the vibration in your skull.

If you feel a bit inhibited about chanting at first, try it when nobody is in the vicinity. The effects are profound, as it induces a wonderful feeling of wellbeing.

Breathing and Relaxation

Relaxation

Relaxation is usually practised after a session of yoga postures and lasts for 15 minutes. You should put on additional warm, loose clothing or cover yourself with a blanket during relaxation, as the body cools down rapidly after exercise and it is difficult to relax when you are cold. You could put on some quiet, gentle music or light a scented candle to enhance the mood.

Yoga relaxation is usually practised in the Pose of the Corpse *(Savasana)*. In this supine posture, your body should be completely still. As your pregnancy advances, you can place a bolster, cushion or folded blanket under your knees to relieve tension in the lower back. As you should not lie on your back for lengthy periods after 30 weeks, you might be more comfortable if you lie on your left side, in the recovery position, with a cushion between your knees.

Relaxing in Savasana

Lie flat on the floor with your body stretched out (use a cushion under your knees if necessary). Have your feet hip distance apart with the toes falling outward. Move your arms slightly away from your body so that there is space in the armpits. Turn your palms up towards the ceiling. Close your eyes and go through the following sequence of actions.

Inhale and point your toes (1), then exhale and relax. Inhale and flex your feet (2), then exhale and relax.

Inhale and pull your buttock muscles so tight that they vibrate against the floor, then exhale and relax. Inhale and push the small of your back into the floor, exhale and relax. Inhale and make tight fists with your hands (3), exhale and relax. Inhale and extend your fingers, hands and arms, until the shoulder blades move away from each other on the floor underneath you (4), then exhale and relax.

Screw up your face and vigorously move your facial muscles around. (This part of the body hardly ever gets exercised, yet it is the one part that we always show to the

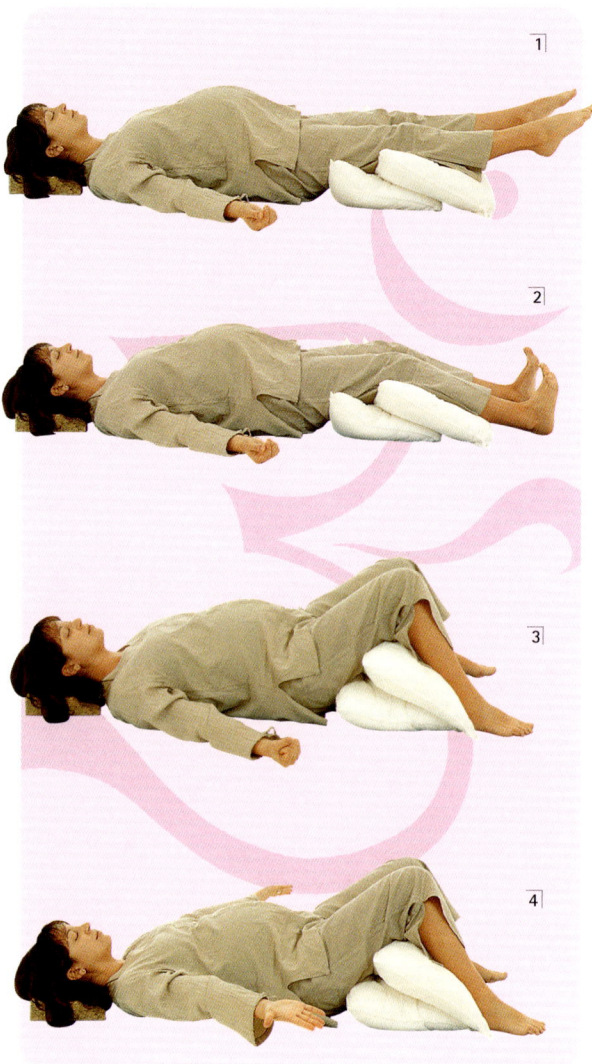

world and never cover.) Relax your face. Gently roll your head from side to side until it feels heavy. Check that you are not clenching your teeth and that your tongue is lying softly in the base of your mouth, not stuck to your palate. Relax your forehead, cheeks and chin.

Do 20 rounds of Ujjayi breathing (see p23) and then allow your body to take on its natural breathing rhythm, moving into a shallower breath. Consciously count the Ujjayi breaths, as this stops the mind from wandering. Lie quietly for the rest of the relaxation period. If you wish to do a visualization (see opposite) now is the time. At the end of the 15 minutes, lightly brush your thumbs across your fingertips and wiggle your toes. Slowly, take your arms up above your head and stretch and yawn. Draw your knees up onto your chest and roll over onto your right side. Lie still for a moment or two with your eyes closed. Then, place your left hand on the floor in front of you and push yourself up into a sitting position. Open your eyes. You should be left with a feeling of languid tranquillity.

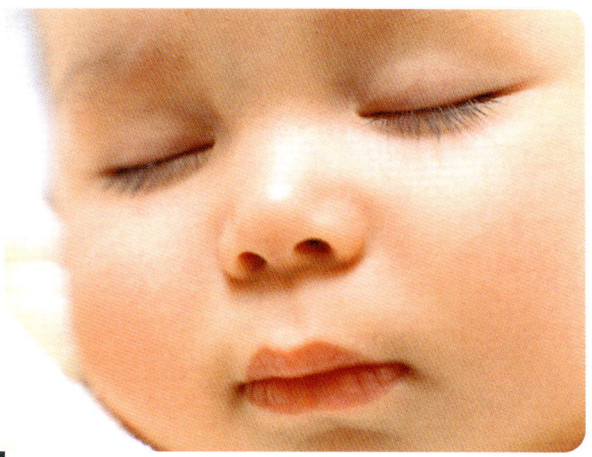

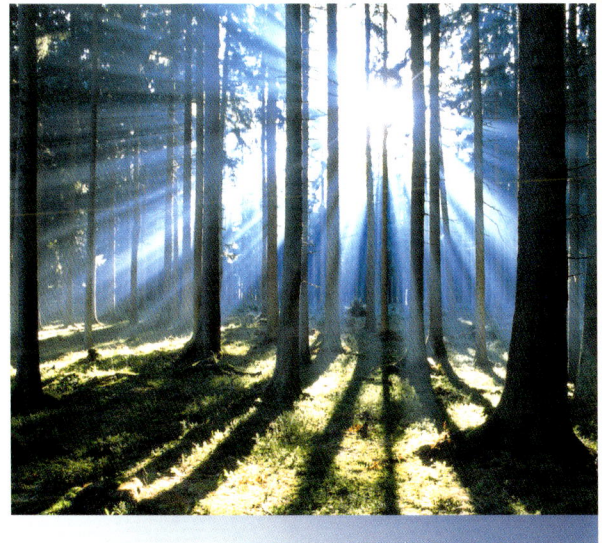

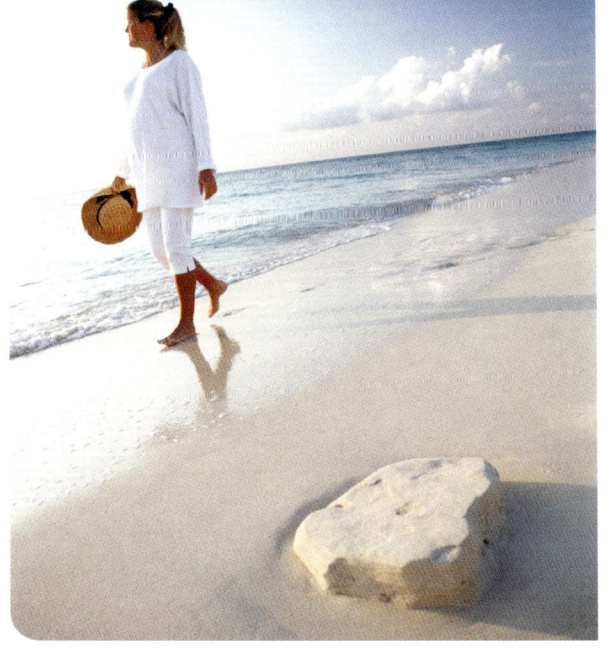

Visualization

Although it might seem difficult to accomplish at first, once you have learned to focus on an image in your mind, visualization is an easy and comfortable exercise which should leave you feeling clear and revitalized.

After the breathing exercises during Savasana, visualize a favourite scene and imagine yourself there. Perhaps you see yourself alone on a deserted beach. See the sun pasted against the blue sky and hear the waves crashing onto the sand. Notice the colour of the sea, the sky and the clouds. Listen to the sound of the ocean and the cry of the gulls. Smell the salt on the air. Picture yourself walking along the sand, picking up shells. The important thing is to bring all your senses into play to create a clear vision in your mind and then try to transport yourself into the scene and see if you can lose yourself in it.

Of course, you do not have to use a beach image. Your chosen scene could be a forest, waterfall or any favourite place, whether actual or imaginary. The important thing is to make the visualization as real as possible by evoking the senses of sight, touch, sound and smell in your mind.

Pregnant women often choose to visualize their unborn child, imagining what it might look like and focusing on its health and wellbeing.

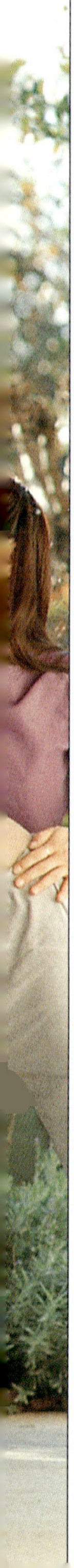

THIS chapter, and the ones that follow, introduce you to a number of postures that are suitable for practising during pregnancy.

This chapter provides some basic information to guide you, whether you practise at home or in a class situation. The next three chapters all follow the same format, starting with the easiest exercises and building up to more advanced postures. If you are new to yoga, it is advisable to start at the beginning of each chapter and work slowly through the exercises until, with progress, you feel each posture becoming easier. Initially you might experience some stiffness or awkwardness while doing the postures but this should soon disappear. Practising a variety of postures will quickly show you which parts of your body are weaker than others and these weaknesses can then gradually be worked on and reduced. You should include a variety of postures in each session, and the sample classes on pp92–93 provide combinations of sitting, standing and supine postures.

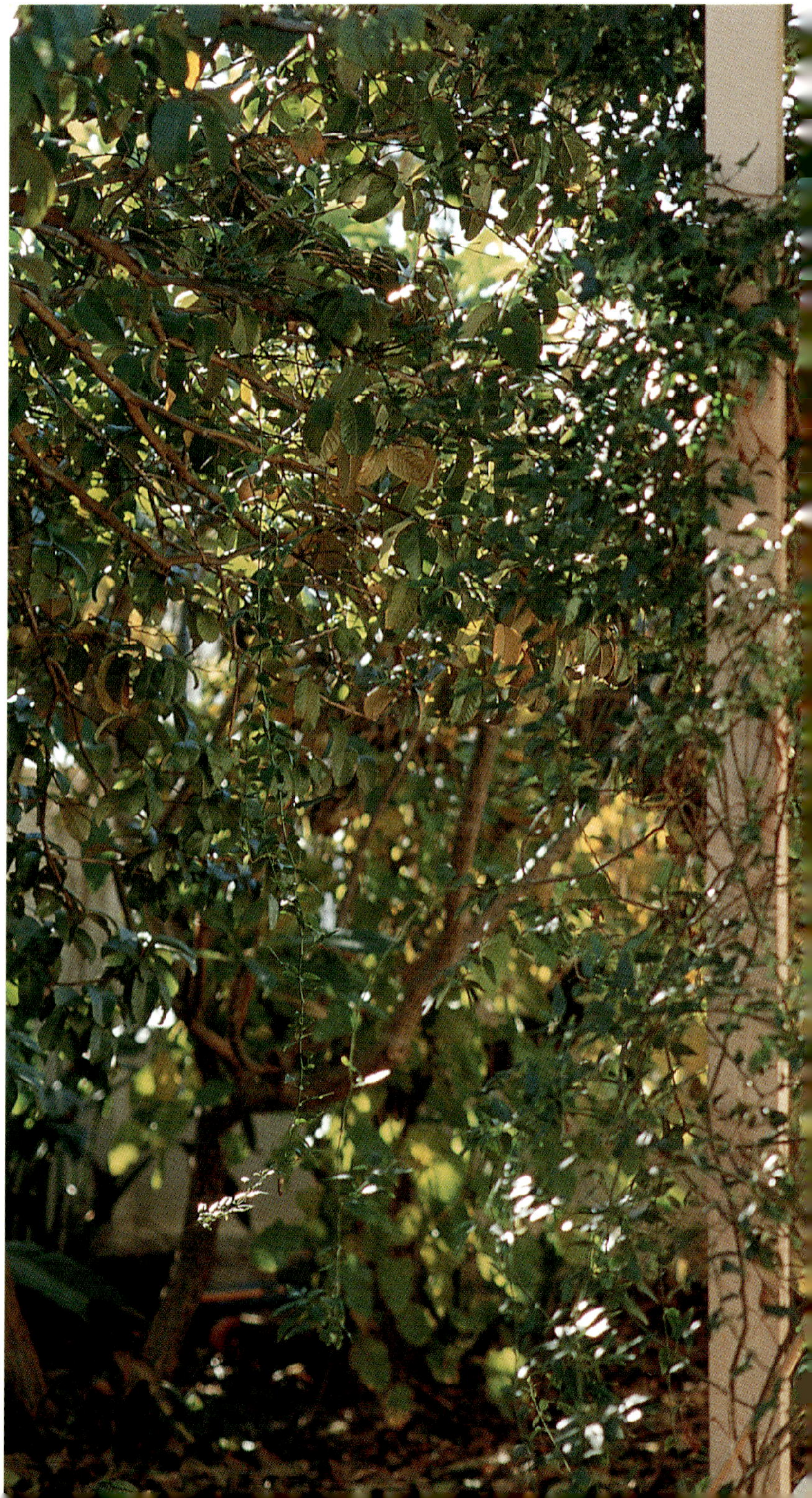

Guidelines For Practice

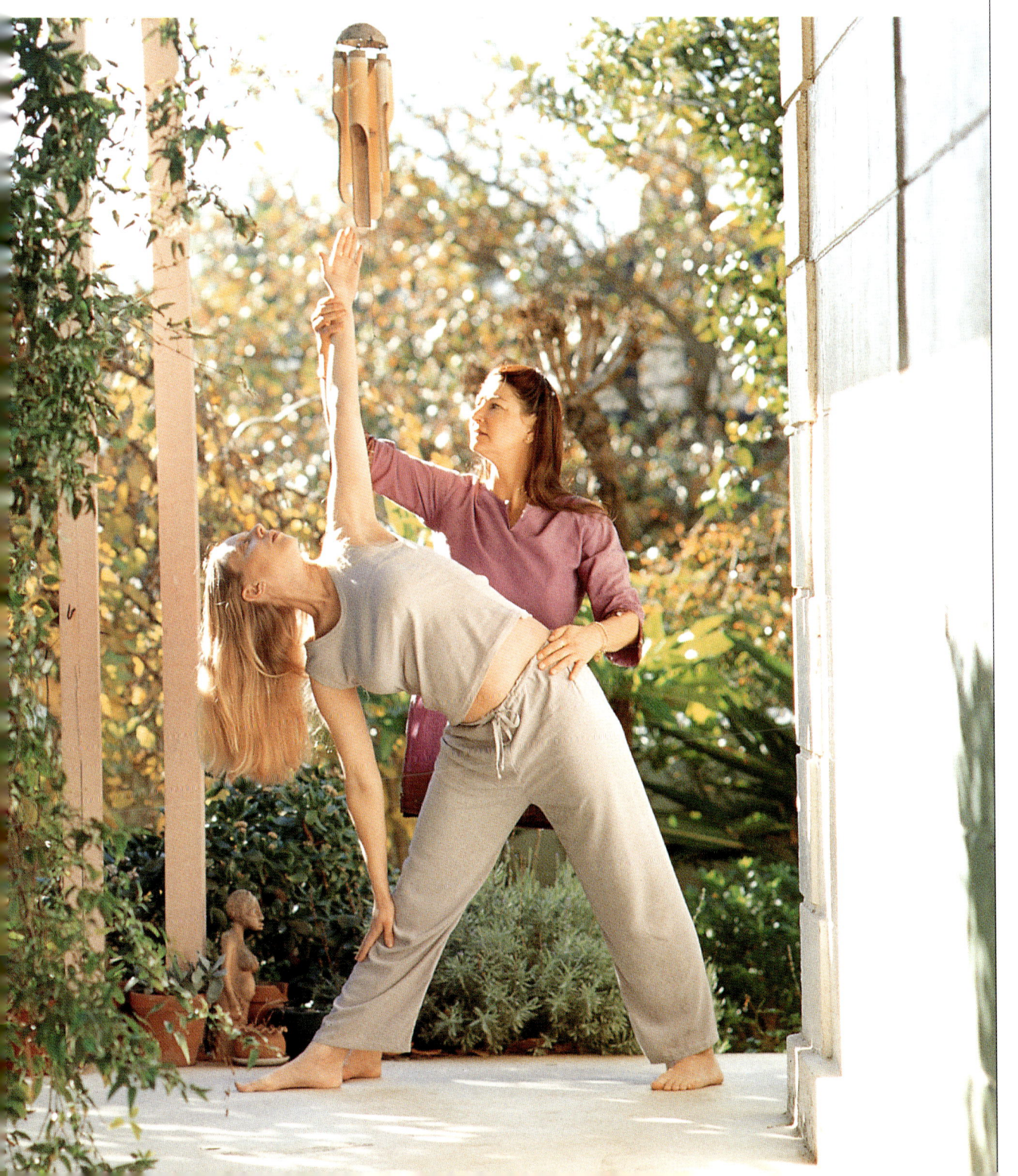

Guidelines for Practice

Yoga should always be pleasurable and comfortable, both physically and mentally. You should not strain, struggle or experience any discomfort or pain during yoga practice. Rather, there should be a sense of extending, flowing and graceful stretching into each pose. Listen to your body at all times. The two main aspects of all yoga postures are steadiness and comfort. Find your comfort zone in a pose and relax into it; do not overextend your muscles. Once the maximum stretch has been attained in a posture, you should be able to hold it for a comfortable period of time. The ability to stretch and relax will be a great help during labour. If you experience any difficulty in attaining a posture, try using a chair, the wall or a partner to carry and balance the bulk of your weight.

Sometimes inner conflict arises when the mind wishes to do more and forgets that the body is not yet ready. If you work your body too hard, it will take its revenge by being stiff and sore the next day.

Try not to let your mind wander during yoga practice. Focus your attention on your breathing and on what your body is doing and how it feels.

In a static posture, such as the Downward-facing Dog Stretch (see p73), the body is held still. In contrast, a dynamic posture, such as the Cat Stretch (see p46), is one in which the body moves. Breathing should remain comfortable in both static and dynamic postures.

Most yoga postures work a certain part of the body quite intensively, so it is necessary to do a counter-posture afterwards to bend the body in an opposite direction, relax your muscles and spine and return your body to a position of symmetry. An example is the Shoulder Stand (see p74), which closes the muscles of the throat and balances the thyroid and parathyroid glands. A counter-posture, such as the Fish (see p57), opens the throat area and allows oxygenated blood to wash over the glands. Rest poses can also be counter-postures.

SOME POINTS TO REMEMBER

- Always work both sides of the body evenly. Whatever you do with one side of the body must be repeated on the other side. (It is normal for one side of the body to be stronger and more flexible than the other.) Work the right side first, then the left, as this aids the natural peristaltic motion of digestion. Almost everything in yoga assists and enhances natural bodily functions.
- Some of the postures in this book have a recommendation as to how many times you should do them. This is not a hard and fast rule. Listen to your body. If you feel like doing more or less than the recommended number, do so.
- Always work with the breath. Each movement should be accompanied by an inhalation or an exhalation. A basic guideline is that when the body lifts or opens, you inhale. This is logical, as there is now space for the lungs to expand. When the body folds or closes, an exhalation helps to squeeze air out of the lungs.
- Never hold your breath or practise breath retention during pregnancy. The foetus requires oxygen at all times.
- It is important to relax between postures to allow the heart rate and breathing to return to normal.
- Keeping your eyes closed will enhance your concentration. (Keep them open during standing postures to help maintain your balance.)
- Your centre of balance changes during pregnancy, so use a wall, chair or a partner to support you when doing inverted or balancing postures.

Points for Practice

- Avoid prone (face-down) postures when your abdomen begins to expand.
- By the third trimester, postures involving lying on your back can cause a drop in blood pressure, as the uterus presses against vessels carrying blood to the placenta. To relax, lie on your side, or place a cushion under one buttock to tilt your back.
- Do not practise inversions in the last trimester, as most babies will already have assumed a head-down position by this stage.
- If you experience pain during any posture, stop immediately and discuss it with your teacher. You may be making a basic error which she will be able to correct. At all times, be gentle with your body. Remember, there are now two lives to consider.
- When doing spinal twists, be careful not to squeeze the enlarged abdomen. Focus the twist in the upper spine, ribs and shoulders.
- Never do a spinal twist straight after a backward bend, or a back bend after a spinal twist. Back bends 'open' the spine and there is a chance that you could pop a disc if you overtwist the spine.
- Do not practise yoga with a full stomach. Allow four hours after a heavy meal and two hours after a light meal before doing yoga. Ensure that the bowel and bladder have been emptied.
- Do not do folded leg postures if you suffer from varicose veins or venous blood clots.
- When bending forward, stretch out from the hips. Do not curve the spine.
- Do not hold your arms above your head if you suffer from high blood pressure.
- Do not clench your teeth while practising your postures. Keep your jaw relaxed.
- Do not force your body to work to the point that it shakes or vibrates. If this occurs, try to relax into the posture or come out of it altogether.
- As your pregnancy progresses it will become more difficult to get up when you have been lying on the floor (see below). The easiest way is to roll onto your right side and place your left hand on the floor (1), using it to push yourself into a sitting position (2). From there, come into a kneeling position and slowly stand up (3).

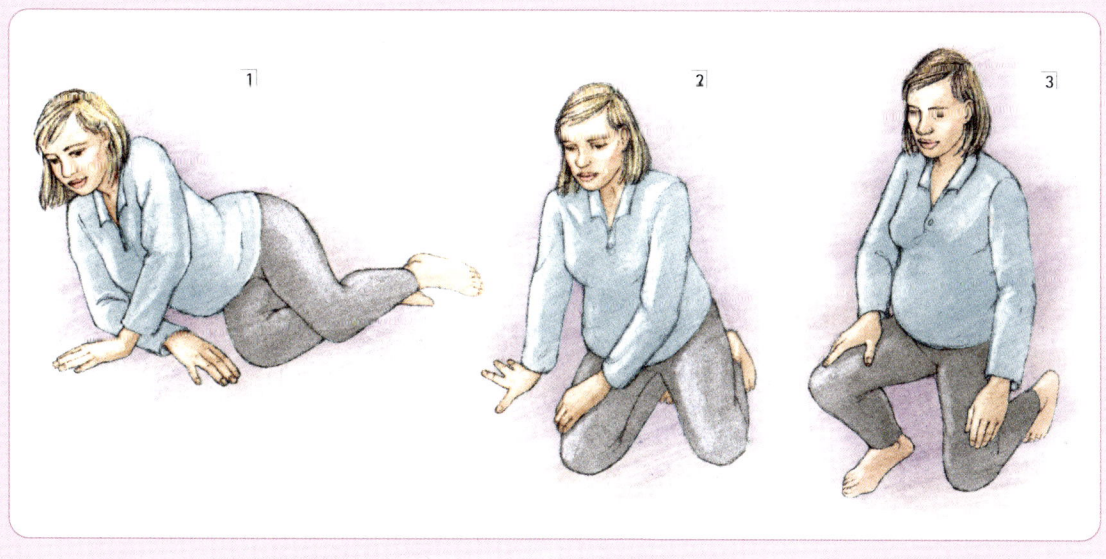

Guidelines for Practice

Attending yoga classes

If you have been practising yoga for some time, it is important to inform your teacher as soon as you know you are pregnant, as certain postures should be avoided during pregnancy. If you have previously had a miscarriage you may need to take extra care in the early weeks. You might even ask to be referred to a teacher who specializes in pregnancy. Teachers who offer classes for pregnant women generally also hold postnatal classes, which help you get back into shape as well as reestablish an exercise routine after birth.

Yoga is most beneficial when it is done regularly. A good teacher will help you to structure your practice by drawing up exercise sessions that can be followed at home. However, attending regular classes is important, as bad habits are easy to pick up, but extremely difficult to break. In class, the teacher will point out your errors and rectify them so that you do not continue making the same mistakes at home.

If you decide to start yoga only after falling pregnant, your healthcare provider, prenatal clinic or maternity goods store may be able to recommend classes or a yoga teacher in your area.

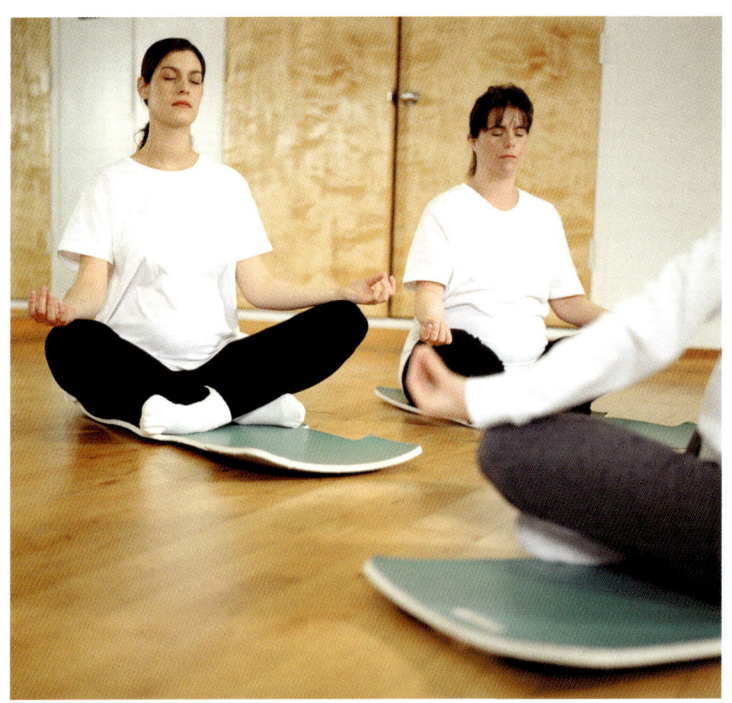

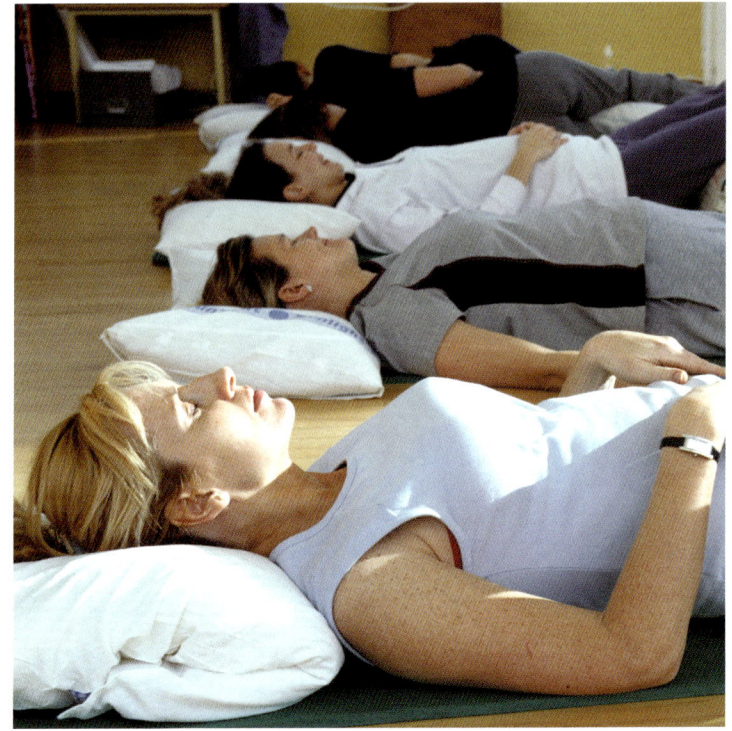

Top right Classes are an opportunity to learn the correct way of doing yoga postures.
Right All yoga sessions should end with a period of relaxation.

Practising at home

Unless you are able to attend three or four classes a week, you will find it beneficial to supplement your classes with sessions at home. You will find it much easier to practise regularly at home if you set aside a specific area, or are able to clear a space with the minimum of effort. There should be enough space for you to stretch out and move with ease. A well-ventilated room that is light, quiet and clean is ideal. Fresh air is preferable, as air conditioning and central heating change the nature of the oxygen we breathe, making it difficult for the body to absorb it. Natural, negatively charged oxygen is beneficial to the body, which is probably why we feel invigorated after a lightning storm. If the weather is pleasant, do your yoga practice outside, wearing as little clothing as decency and the temperature permit.

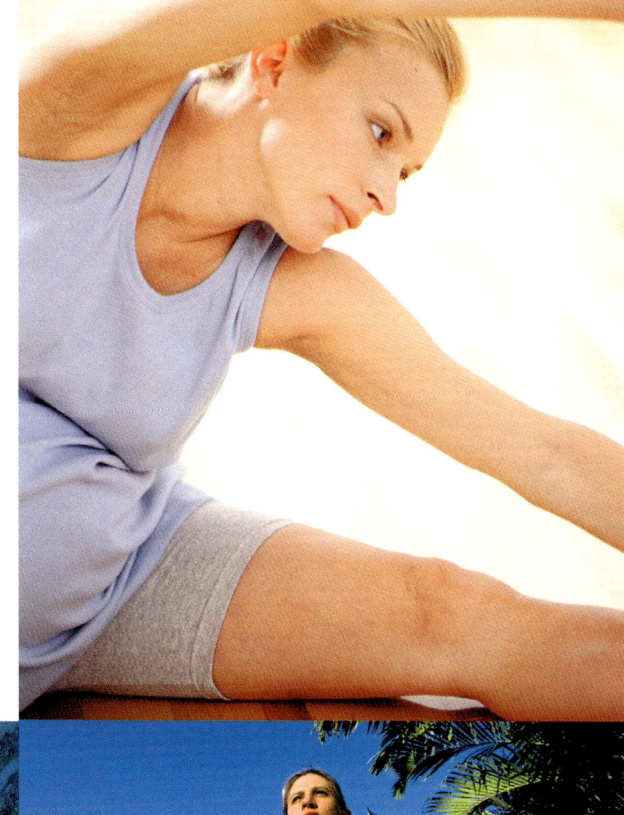

Above Make the most of fine weather by exercising outdoors, taking advantage of fresh air and sunshine.

Top Clear enough floor space to allow you to move freely.

Left Exercising in water is a wonderful way to limber up before a yoga session. It also soothes aching muscles.

Guidelines for Practice

Clothing

Our bodies are less supple in the morning than in the evening, but a warm shower can help to loosen your muscles and joints before a morning yoga session. Whatever time of day you choose, try to ensure that you will not be interrupted. Lock the door if necessary, and disconnect the phone or turn on the answering machine.

A yoga class usually consists of one hour of exercises and breathing followed by 15 minutes of relaxation. If you cannot manage an hour at home, or feel that it will be too much for your body, then do as much as you are comfortable with. However, it is essential to relax after each exercise session as this enables the body to absorb the benefit of the exercises it has just completed.

It is essential for a pregnant woman to learn how to consciously relax so that she will be able to 'let go' between each contraction during labour. Finish your yoga session at home with a period of relaxation in Savasana (see p26), with or without Ujjayi breathing.

You might choose to play some gentle background music, either for the duration of the entire yoga session or just while you relax.

It is not necessary to buy special clothing for yoga, and your degree of pregnancy will often dictate your choice of clothing. Most practitioners choose leggings or loose elasticized trousers, worn together with a leotard, conventional T-shirt, flowing top, or a close-fitting sports vest or crop-top.

Whatever you wear, choose items that are cool, comfortable and do not restrict your movements in any way. Avoid garments that will flop over your face when you bend forward or do inverted postures. In cold weather, begin by wearing a layer of warm clothing, taking off items as your body warms up, and putting them back on if you feel yourself starting to get cold.

Although bare feet are preferable for yoga practice, you can wear socks if the weather is cold, or until your body and feet are warmed up.

If possible, exercise in front of a full-length mirror, as this will help you to check your position in the postures.

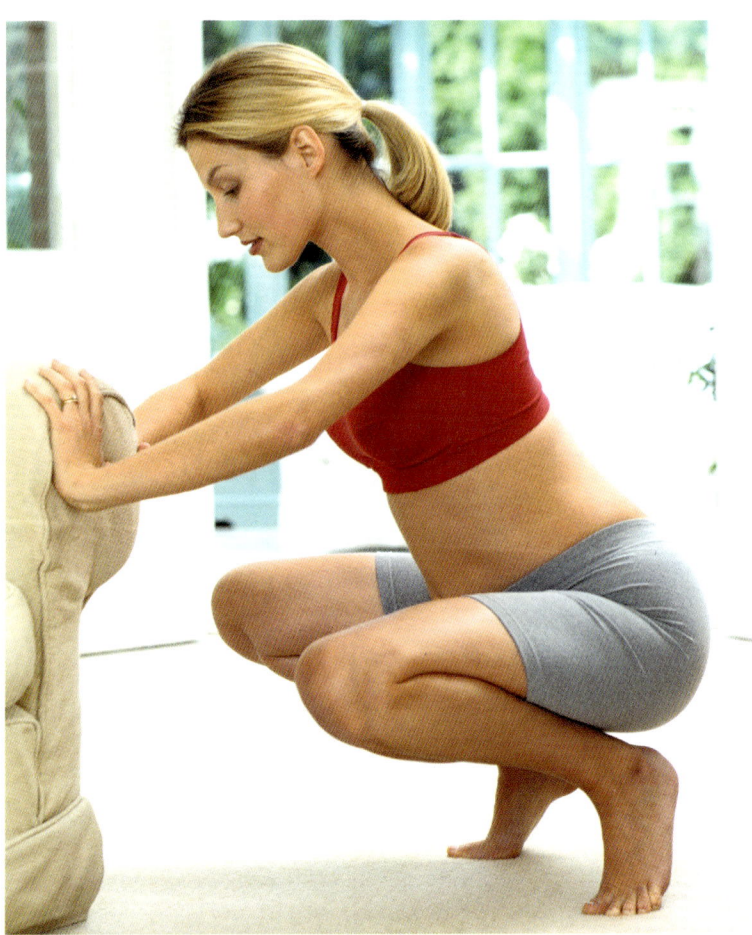

Right When you exercise at home, use furniture to provide balance or support for various postures.

Yoga Equipment

Equipment

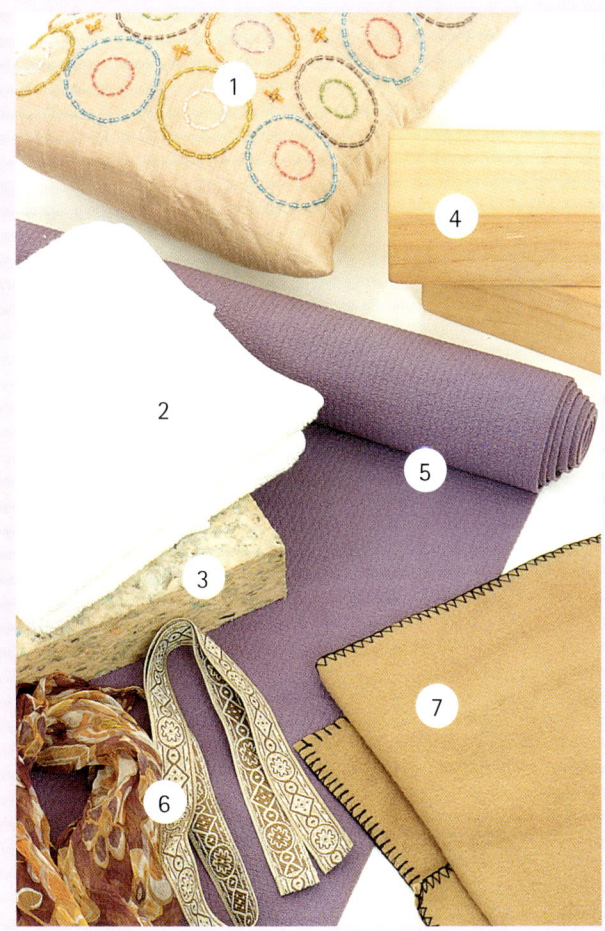

Special non-slip yoga mats are available to place on the floor or on the ground, but they are not essential. A large bath towel or small rug will suffice, provided it will not slide around. Bolsters, cushions or pillows and a sturdy upright chair can be used for support in the more difficult postures, while a long strap (at least 1m, or 3.5ft, long), belt or folded towel may help you to reach and hold your feet in certain postures.

Ensure that whatever items you require are close at hand before you start an exercise session.

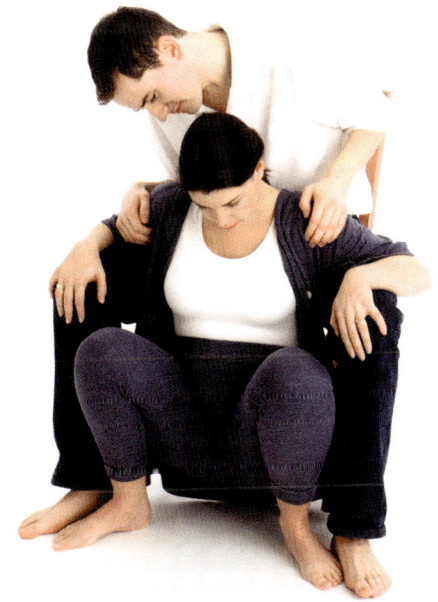

Above Use a cushion or pillow (1), towel (2) or special yoga sponge (3) under your knees when lying on your back. Place wooden blocks (4) under your heels when doing squats and knee bends. A non-slip yoga mat (5) works best on a smooth surface. Belts, straps or scarves (6) help extend your reach.

Above right The supported squat is a popular birth position. Practise it with your partner beforehand.

Right A blanket (7) will keep you warm during relaxation.

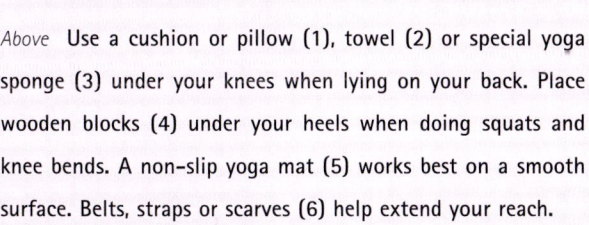

35

Sitting postures calm the mind, soothe the nerves, relieve fatigue and promote sleep. They can be divided into forward bends, backbends and spinal twists. Sitting forward bends benefit the navel chakra, which relates to the kidneys and adrenal glands (see p15), so practising them helps to balance and strengthen these organs. Sitting forward bends are also a good preparation for standing forward bends. If you suffer from high blood pressure or a heart condition, you should always choose the sitting version over the standing option when doing forward bends.

Supine (or lying down) postures open the groin, increase flexibility in the spine and strengthen the back, arms and legs.

> A simple graphic indicates whether a posture is suitable for:
> BEGINNERS (B | 1 2 3)
> INTERMEDIATE (I | 1 2 3)
> or ADVANCED (A | 1 2 3)
> practitioners, and whether it is safe to practise in the first, second or third trimester. However, you should take into account your own level of fitness and yoga experience, as well as your medical practitioner's advice. Work within your own limits and never force your body beyond its comfort zone.

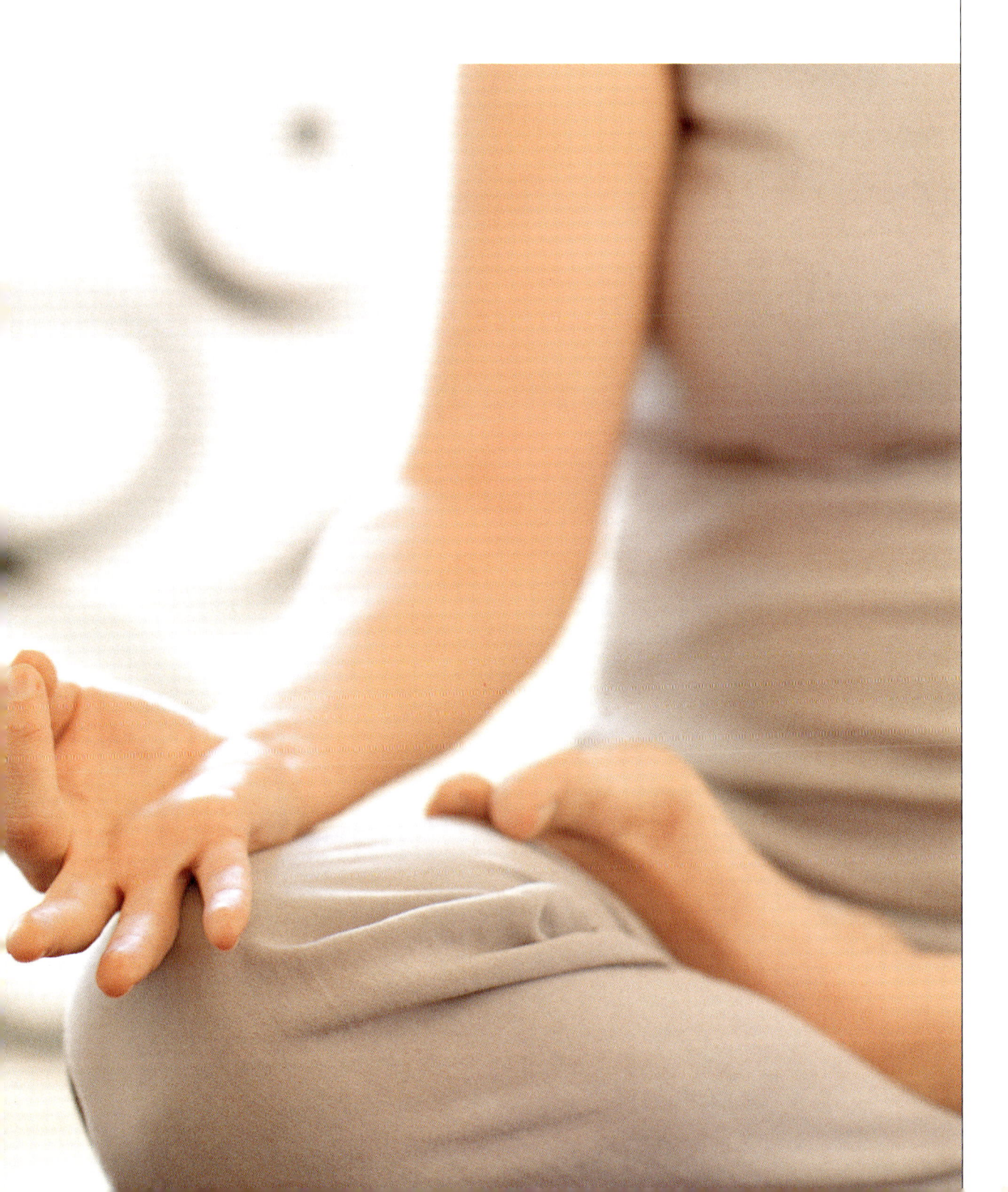

Sitting and Supine Postures

Sitting and Supine Postures

NECK RELEASES
B 1 2 3

BENEFITS Releases tension in the neck and at the top of the shoulders.
CAUTIONS Ensure that your shoulders do not pull upwards. Keep them well stretched down towards the floor. Do these neck exercises as slowly as your breathing enables you to.
METHOD Sit on the floor in a position that you find most comfortable (see pp41 and 43 for two classic positions). Take a preparatory Ujjayi breath, in and out (see p23). Keep the Ujjayi breath going for the duration of each part of this exercise.

A: Inhale and on the exhalation slowly bring your chin down onto your chest. (1). The length of time that it takes to drop the chin as low as possible should equal the length of the exhalation. On the inhalation slowly raise your head back to its natural position (2). On the next exhalation raise your chin up towards the ceiling and extend the muscles of the throat upwards (3). Open and close your mouth wide three times while the chin is pointed upwards. Bring your head back to its natural position on the inhalation. Repeat the entire exercise three times.

B: Inhale and stretch your left arm away from your body at a 45-degree angle. As you exhale, bend your neck, bringing your right ear to your right shoulder, pressing both shoulders down towards the floor (1). Inhale and bring your head to its natural position. Repeat this three times. On the third exhalation lower your left arm to your side. Repeat with your right arm stretched, lowering your left ear (2).

These exercises flow in sequence. The first releases tension from the back of the neck and the throat area, while the second releases tension from the sides of the neck.

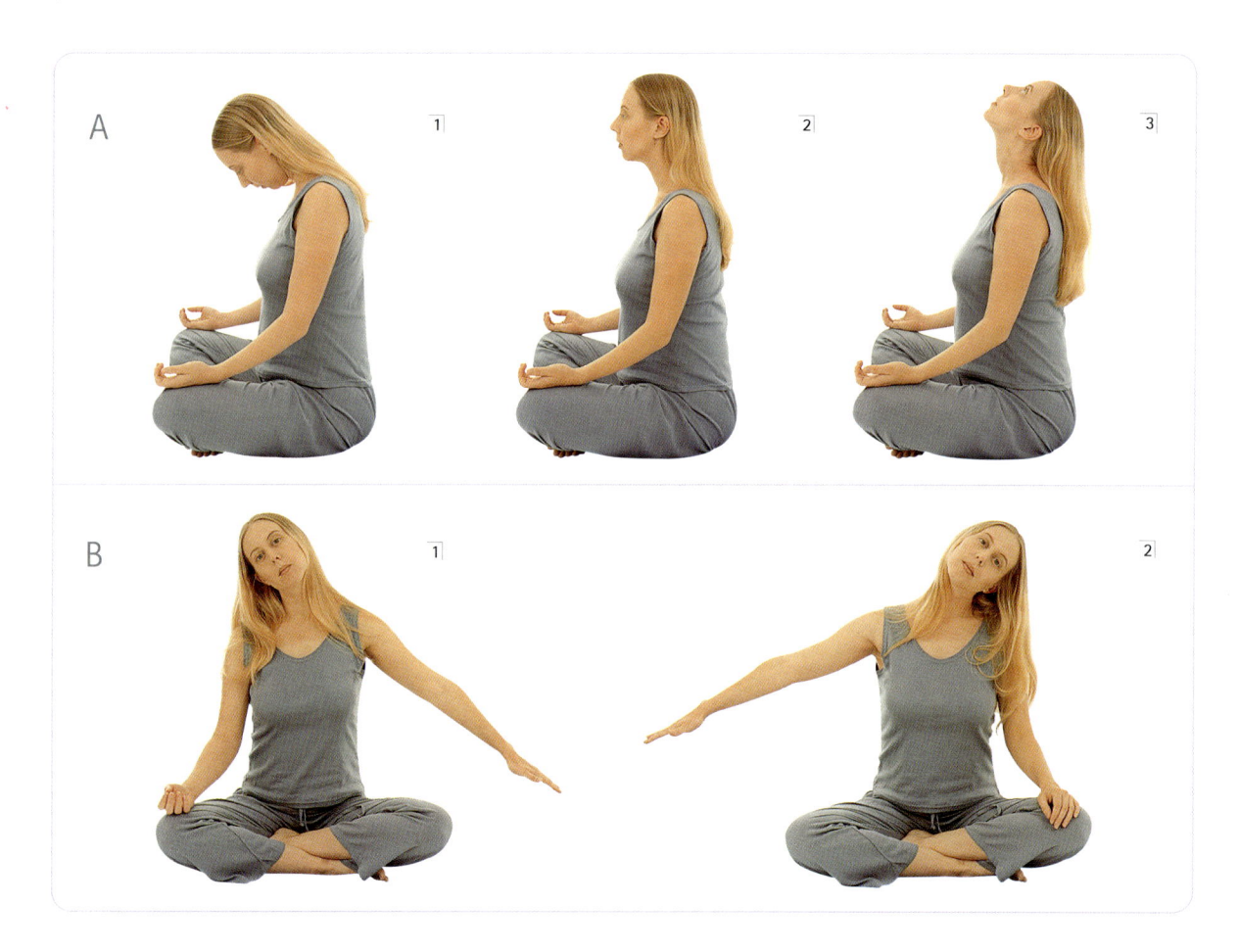

SHOULDER ROLLS

(B | 1 2 3)

BENEFITS Releases tension in the shoulders.

METHOD Sit in a position that is comfortable for you. Take a preparatory Ujjayi breath in and out. On the next inhalation push the shoulders slowly forwards and then bring them up towards the ceiling (2). As you exhale, draw the shoulder blades together behind you (3) and then pull them down towards the floor (4). It should feel as though you are making a large, slow circle with your shoulders. Repeat the entire exercise three times. Now do the same exercise four times in the other direction, so that the shoulder blades are first drawn backwards and then upwards on the inhalation. Roll the shoulders forwards and then bring them back down towards the floor on the exhalation.

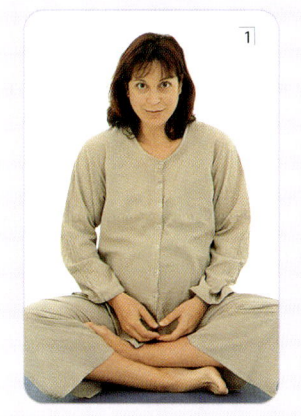

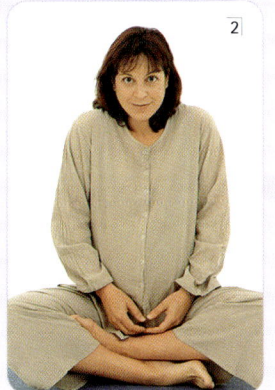

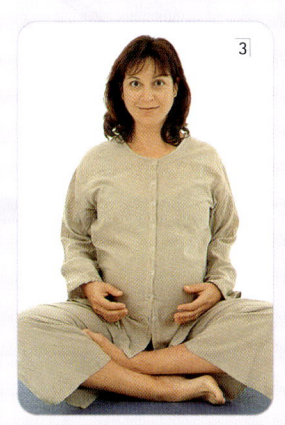

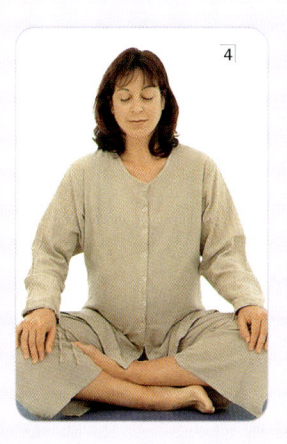

APANASANA

(This posture, which has no direct English name, is often referred to as the wind-relieving posture.)

(B | 1 2)

BENEFITS Assists in removing all toxins (apana) from the body. Apanasana helps to remove carbon dioxide from the lungs and aids digestion and elimination, as it massages the internal abdominal organs. It is an excellent posture for women who suffer from menstrual problems as it soothes cramps and aids the blood flow. However, it is perfectly safe for pregnant women, who should practise the open-legged version shown here. This exercise also alleviates backache. This easy, but important, yoga posture is used as a counter-position for many postures involving the legs and hips. It should be very comforting to do.

METHOD Lie on your back and draw your knees up onto your chest (knees open and feet together). Place your right hand on your right knee and your left hand on your left knee. Keep your hands on your knees for the duration of the exercise. As you inhale, straighten your elbows and allow your knees to slowly move away from you. As you exhale, draw your knees slowly down onto your chest. Repeat this 10 to 20 times. Make sure that your buttocks stay in contact with the floor at all times. As with all yoga postures, practise the Ujjayi breath while doing this exercise. If you suffer from general lower back pain, push the small of the back firmly into the floor as you hug your knees towards your chest.

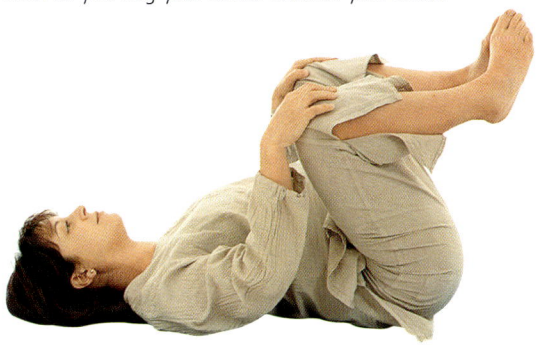

Sitting and Supine Postures

Pose of the Child
Balasana

B | 1 2 3

BENEFITS This is an extremely calming and soothing posture and is mostly used as a rest position in-between more difficult poses.
METHOD Sit on your knees and lean forward to rest your forehead on the floor. Allow your arms to relax on the floor next to your body with your hands next to your feet. Your shoulder blades should feel as if they are moving away from each other and your back is becoming broader. Allow your shoulders to fall down towards the floor. Relax into the pose and breathe gently and evenly.

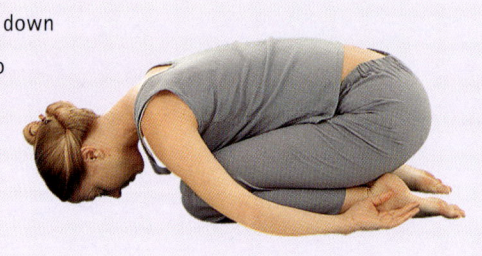

VARIATION As your pregnancy develops it will become necessary to open your knees to allow space for the expanding abdomen. If you are not one hundred per cent comfortable in this posture make your hands into fists and place them on top of each other, then rest your forehead on top of your fists.

The Frog
Mandukasana

B | 1 2 3

BENEFITS Stretches the hips and the inner thigh muscles.
CAUTIONS If the stretch on the inner thighs is too intense, then bring the knees a little closer together. If you cannot feel the stretch, take the knees wider apart.
METHOD Sit on your knees and open them to a comfortably wide position (1). Let your big toes touch each other underneath your buttocks. Place your hands on the floor between the knees (2), inhale and lift your sternum (breastbone), keeping your spine straight. As you exhale, walk your hands forwards until your chest is resting on the floor (3). Try not to lift your buttocks off your heels. If possible, place your forehead on the floor. If you feel very comfortable in this pose, try placing your chin on the floor for a more intense stretch. Hold the posture for as long as it is comfortable, while practising the Ujjayi breath.

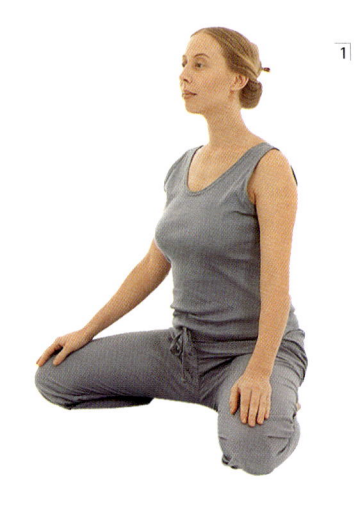

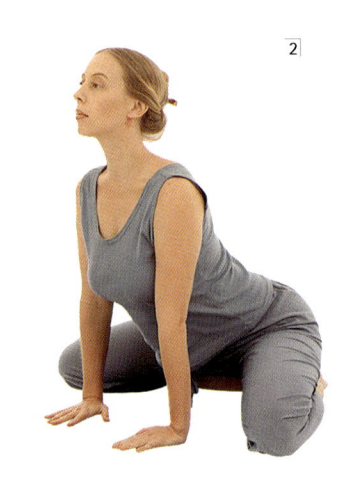

40

The Pelvic Uplift

Mula Bandha

B 1 2 3

BENEFITS This is probably one of the most beneficial exercises you can do during pregnancy, so do not neglect it. It strengthens the perineum and the pelvic floor and will help you to control and relax the pelvic muscles during birth. It can also assist with incontinence and prolapse of the uterus (when uterus sinks from its normal position). You can practise the pelvic uplift anywhere, at any time, not only during a yoga session.

CAUTION If you suffer from haemorrhoids, practise this posture on all fours with your buttocks in the air and your head down.

METHOD Sit in a comfortable position. Inhale and draw the anal, rectal and pelvic muscles upwards as though you are desperate to go to the toilet but can't find one. Keep drawing the muscles upwards as you exhale. Inhale, then slowly release the muscles as you exhale. Repeat this six times. With practice, you should be able to hold the posture for as long as six or seven breaths. When you get used to the feeling of this exercise try to release the muscles in three stages. First release the outer anal muscles, then the inner rectal muscles and finally the pelvic floor muscles.

The Comfortable Position

Sidhasana

B 1 2 3

BENEFITS This exercise brings about flexibility in the hip joints and shoulders.

METHOD Sit in an upright position and draw your left heel in towards the perineum. Bend your right knee and place your right foot in front of the left one (1). Inhale. As you exhale, walk your hands away from you, bringing your chest and head down towards the floor (2). Try to maintain contact between your left buttock and the floor. Straighten your elbows if possible, as this will give a deeper stretch into the shoulders (3). Keep your spine straight. You should feel a stretch in your right hip joint. Hold the position for as long as it feels comfortable and then walk your hands back towards you on an inhalation, so that you come up into a sitting position. Change your legs over so that the left foot is now in front of the right one and do the exercise again. This will work your left hip.

COUNTER-POSTURE Stretch your legs out in front of you and move your feet slowly from side to side. This should release any tension that might have built up in the hip area.

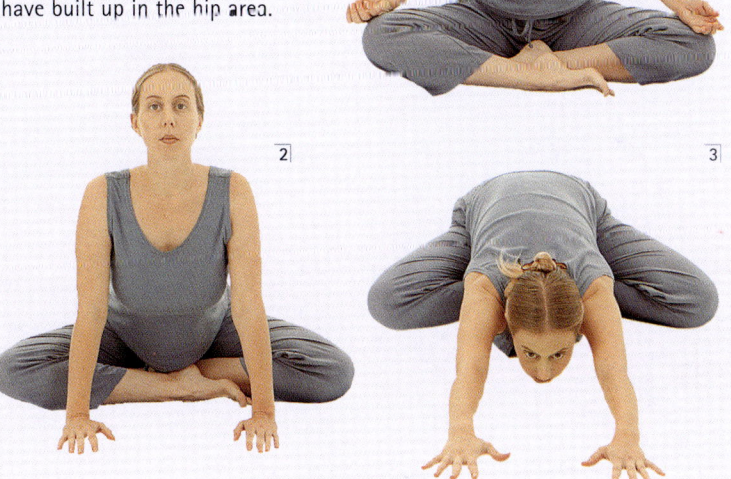

Sitting and Supine Postures

The Cobbler's Pose
Butterfly Pose

Baddha Konasana

 B | 1 2 3

BENEFITS Stretches the hips, pelvis and inner thigh muscles.

METHOD Sit in an upright position, with the soles of your feet touching each other and the heels as close to the perineum as possible (1). Lift your sternum to straighten your spine, and relax your shoulders. Make gentle butterfly movements with your knees, trying to get them as close to the ground as possible (2). For a more intense stretch in the hips, extend your torso and head forwards without bending the spine (3). This is an excellent position in which to practise the pelvic uplift.

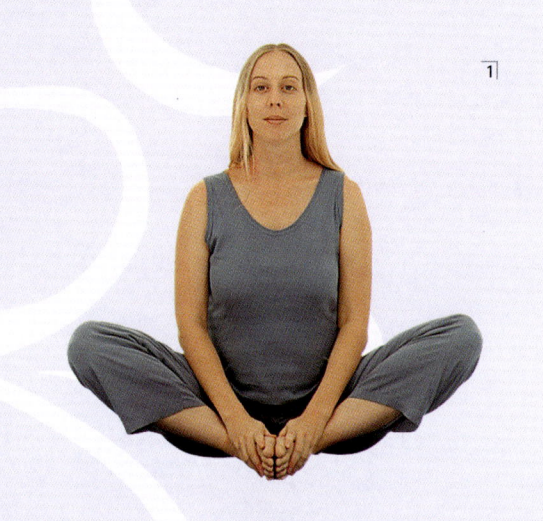

VARIATION

 B | 1 2

CAUTION Do not do this after 30 weeks.

Sit against a wall with your right hip touching it. Lean back on your left elbow and swivel your back so that your body is at right angles to the wall and your legs are against it. Lie back with your head on the floor (or a cushion) and bend your knees, drawing your heels close to the perineum, with the soles of the feet touching. Try to press your knees against the wall.

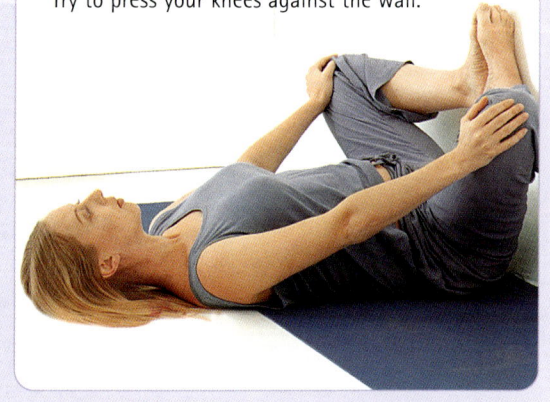

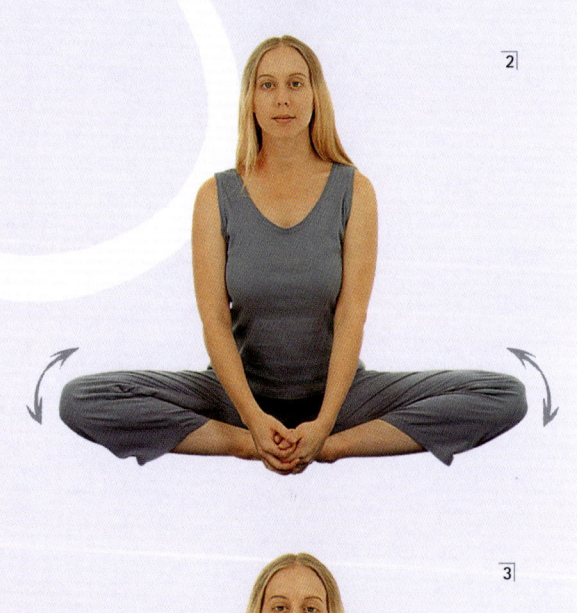

42

The Lotus

Padmasana

(A | 1 | 2 | 3)

BENEFITS Brings flexibility to the hips and pelvic area and develops a straight spine. This classic yoga posture is frequently used in meditation.

CAUTION Knees. Do not attempt the Lotus (Padmasana) until you are fully comfortable with Sidhasana (see p41).

METHOD Sit on your mat with your legs stretched out in front of you. Take hold of your right foot in both hands and draw it up towards your nose. Do not take your nose down towards your toes. Once the foot is lifted, place it as high up the left thigh as possible (1). In fact, try to place your foot on the inside of your left hipbone, as this will avoid pushing the thigh muscle into the bone. Not everybody can do this, but if you can you will find the posture more comfortable. Gently push your right knee as close to the floor as possible with your hand.

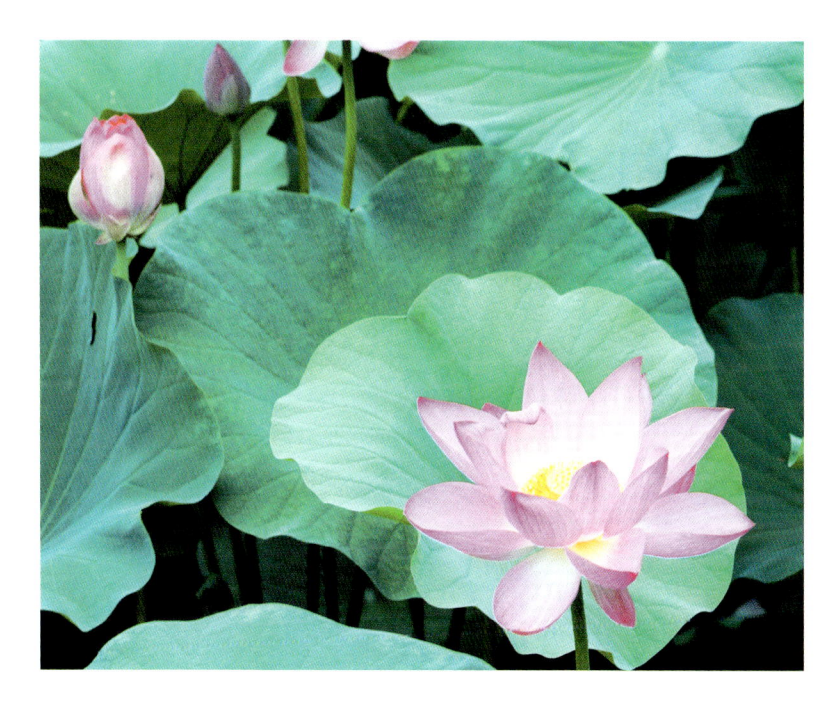

Now, take hold of your left foot with both hands and fold it up on top of your right thigh (2). Hold the posture for as long as it is comfortable. If you cannot get your left foot onto the thigh, just rest it on the floor in front of your right knee (3). (This is known as the Half Lotus.)

If you are very comfortable in the Lotus, close your eyes and practise deep breathing. This is another good position in which to practise the Pelvic Uplift (see p41).

To come out of the posture, unlock your legs, stretch them out in front of you and give them a good shake.

Repeat the exercise, this time bring your left foot up onto your right thigh first, then place your right foot on top of your left thigh.

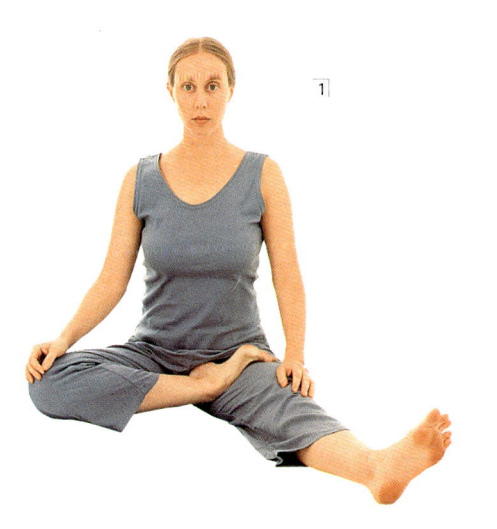

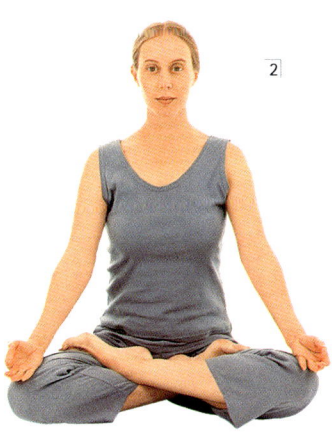

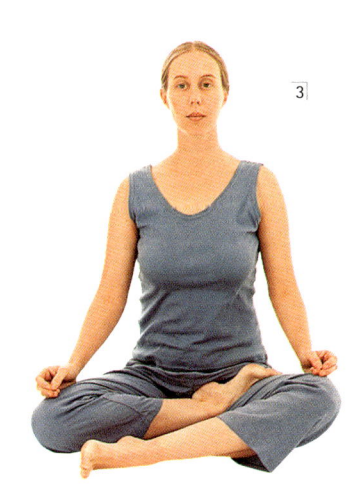

Sitting and Supine Postures

The Baby
B 1 2

BENEFITS Stretches open the hips and the pelvic area.

CAUTIONS Should not be done after 30 weeks.

METHOD Lie on your back and draw your knees onto your chest (1). Keeping your knees bent, raise your feet to the ceiling so that your shins are perpendicular to the floor (2). Take hold of the outer edges of your feet with your hands and draw your knees straight down towards the armpits (3). Press your tailbone into the floor. Hold the position for as long as it is comfortable and then place your feet back on the floor with your knees bent.

COUNTER-POSTURE Keeping your knees bent, inhale and, as you exhale, drop both knees over your right side so that they touch the floor. Do not lift your feet up. Inhale and return your knees to the starting position. As you exhale, take your knees over to the floor on the left. Inhale and raise your knees back to the centre. Repeat this five times to each side. Dropping your knees from side to side should release any tension that might have built up in the hip area during the main posture.

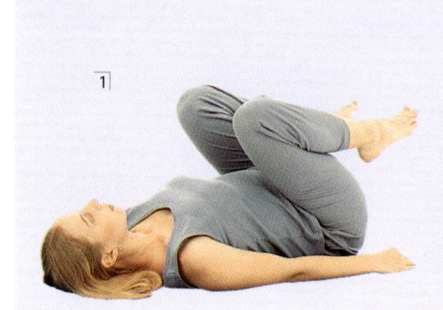

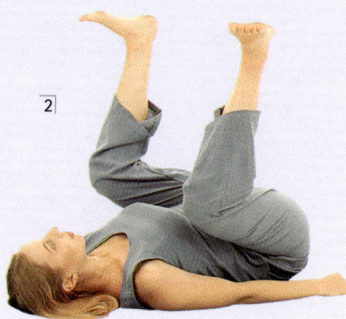

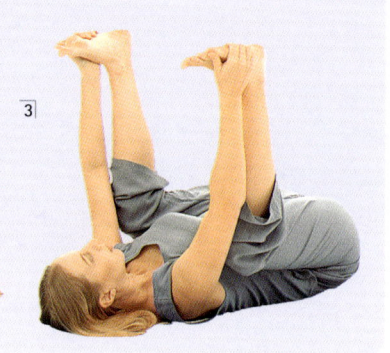

Pelvic Tilt
B 1 2

BENEFITS This subtle posture is excellent for releasing tension from the lower back.

METHOD Lie flat on your mat and bend your knees so that your heels are close to your buttocks. Have your feet hip distance apart and parallel to each other. Exhale and gently push the small of your back into the floor (1). Your tailbone should lift just a little way off the floor. As you inhale, slowly rock onto your tailbone, lifting your navel up towards the ceiling. There should now be a little space between the small of your back and the floor (2). (Note: the arms normally lie next to the body, but in order to demonstrate the movement, the model has moved her arms to the side.)

This is a dynamic exercise, so do it 10 more times, moving slowly with the rhythm of your breathing. You should not experience any discomfort in your back. Although it is a small movement, it releases tension in the lumbar area and can help to relieve backache.

COUNTER-POSTURE Apanasana (see p39).

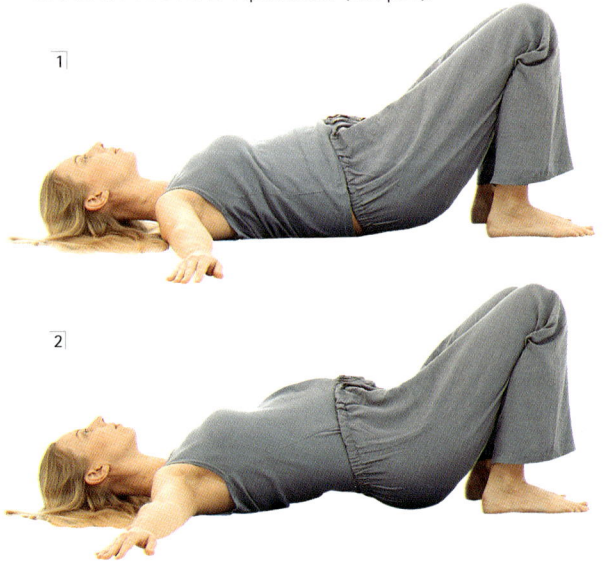

THE HERO

Virasana

(1 | 2 3)

BENEFITS Opens the heart and lung area, and stretches the thighs and the ligaments in the knees.

CAUTIONS Not advised if you suffer from knee problems or are experiencing swollen legs. If you suffer from high blood pressure, do not raise your hands above your head; instead, place them in the prayer position with your thumbs touching your sternum. Ensure that you do not pull your shoulders up underneath the ears during Virasana.

METHOD Sit on your heels with your feet a little apart and your knees close together. Lower your buttocks into the space between your feet (1). It may be necessary to place a cushion or foam block under your buttocks as this is an intense stretch in the thigh area (see below). Inhale and raise your arms above your head. Interlace your fingers and, as you exhale, turn your palms up towards the ceiling (2). Drop your shoulders to release any tension in them. Ensure that your elbows are straight. Practice Ujjayi breathing and hold the posture for as long as it is comfortable. When you have had enough, slowly lower your arms sideways towards the floor on an exhalation and unlock your legs.

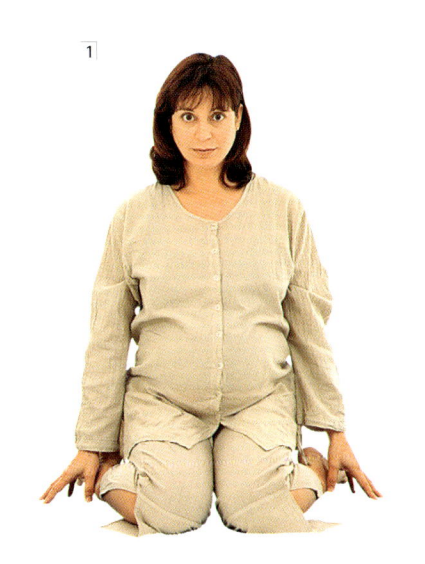

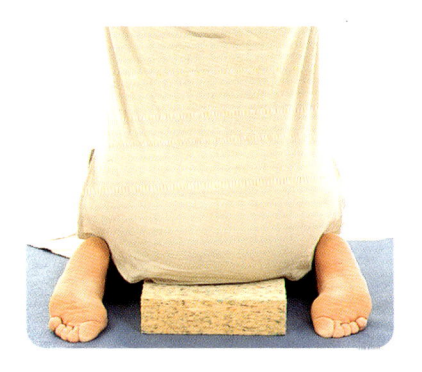

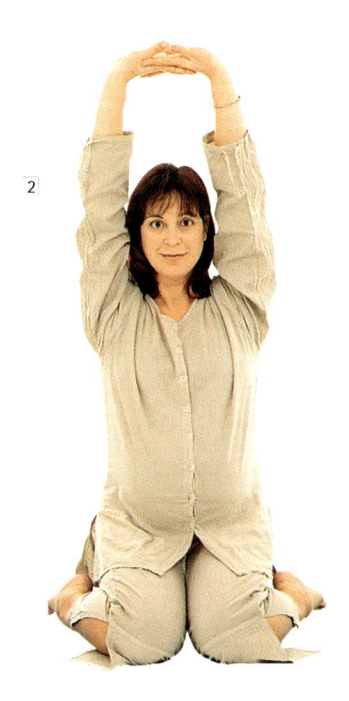

COUNTER-POSTURE Stretch your legs out and give them a vigorous shake.

VARIATION

RECLINING HERO POSTURE

Supta Virasana

(A | 1 2)

CAUTIONS Knees and lower back; high blood pressure.

METHOD Sit as for the Hero posture. Place your hands on the floor next to your feet and slowly lower yourself backwards onto your elbows, bringing your upper back and the back of your head into contact with the floor. As you lie back it might be necessary to bring your elbows closer to your feet. Release your weight from your elbows and take your hands onto the floor above your head in the prayer position.

This is a strong posture which requires experience. When first practising it, it might be wise to place a cushion or folded blanket under your spine.

Sitting and Supine Postures

Cat Stretch and Cat Stretch Balances
Bidalasana

B 1 2 3

BENEFITS Enhances the spine's flexibility. The variations will also increase your balance, improve concentration and are very calming. The extended Cat Stretch stretches the shoulders.

METHOD Kneel on all fours. Place your hands directly underneath your shoulders with your fingers spread wide and the middle fingers parallel to each other. Make sure your knees are directly underneath your hips, hip distance apart (1). Take a preparatory Ujjayi breath (inhalation and exhalation). On the next inhalation, slowly raise your chest and head (2), keeping your spine level. It should feel as though you are trying to touch your spine with the back of your head. The slow movement should match the length of the inhalation.

As you exhale, slowly drop your tailbone and arch your back up towards the ceiling. Drop your head, as though you were trying to see your navel. Push down firmly on your hands and knees (3). This movement should last for the same length of time as the exhalation.

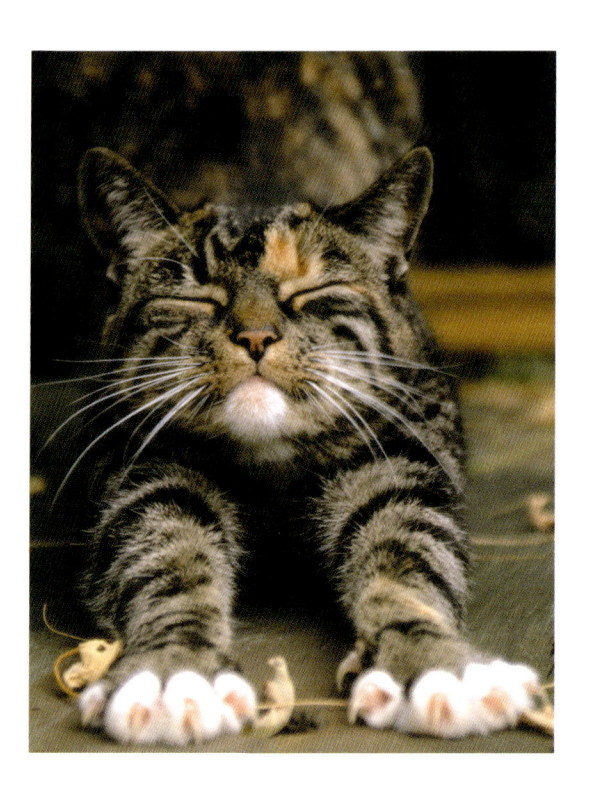

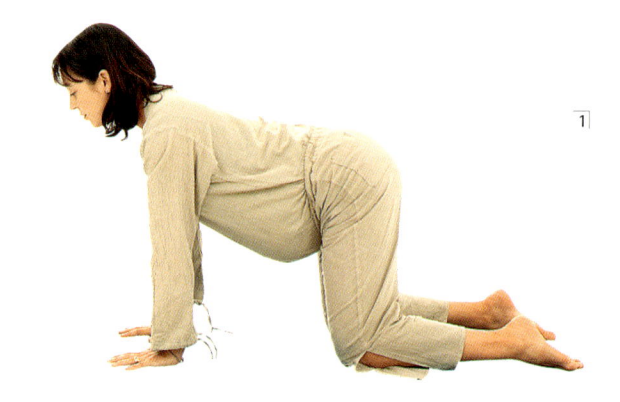

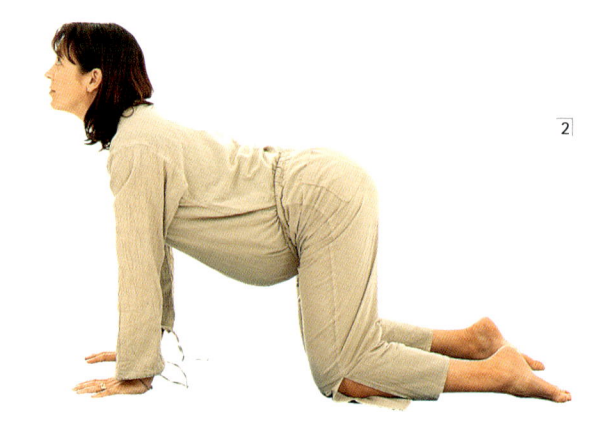

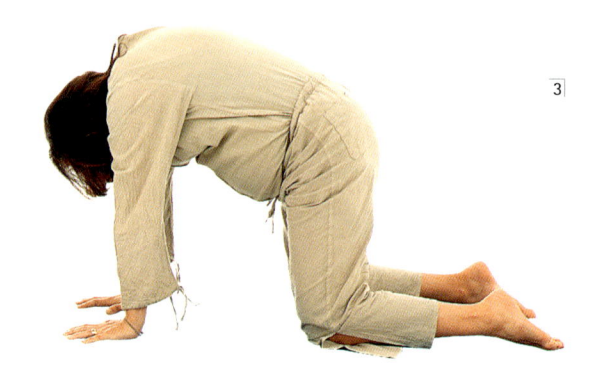

Repeat the Cat Stretch exercise seven times, ensuring that the movement along your spine remains very smooth and controlled, not jerky.

COUNTER-POSTURE Pose of the Child (see p40).

Cat Stretch

VARIATION 1

Cat Stretch Balances
(1 | 1 2 3)

METHOD As with the cat stretch, start on all fours with your hands and knees in the same position (1). Raise your left leg and stretch into your heel. Point your toes down towards the floor, push your heel away from you and drop your left hip towards the floor. When you are steady, raise your right arm (2). Ensure that you keep breathing and that you are not holding your breath. Hold the posture for as long as it is comfortable. Return your hand and knee to the starting position and take a recovery breath. Repeat with your right leg and left arm.

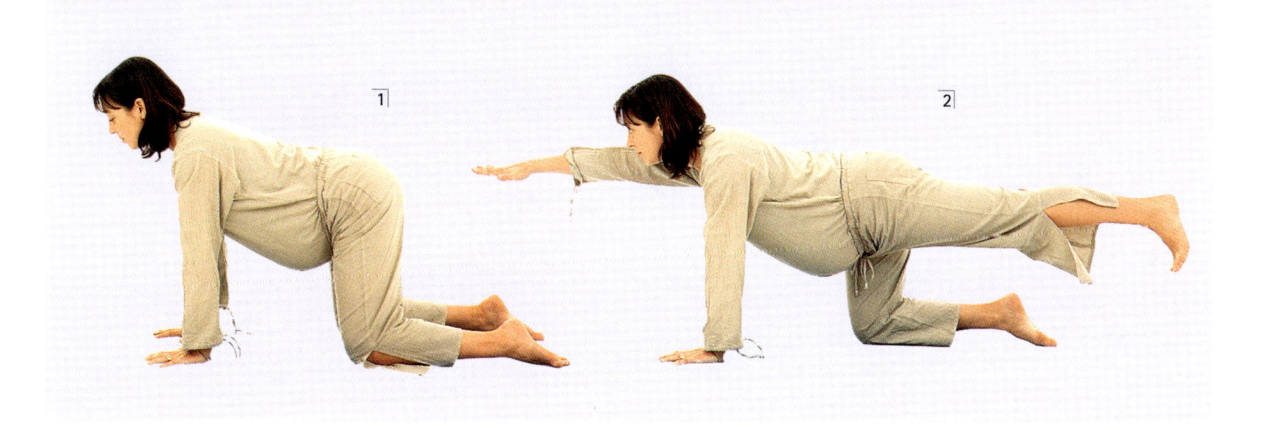

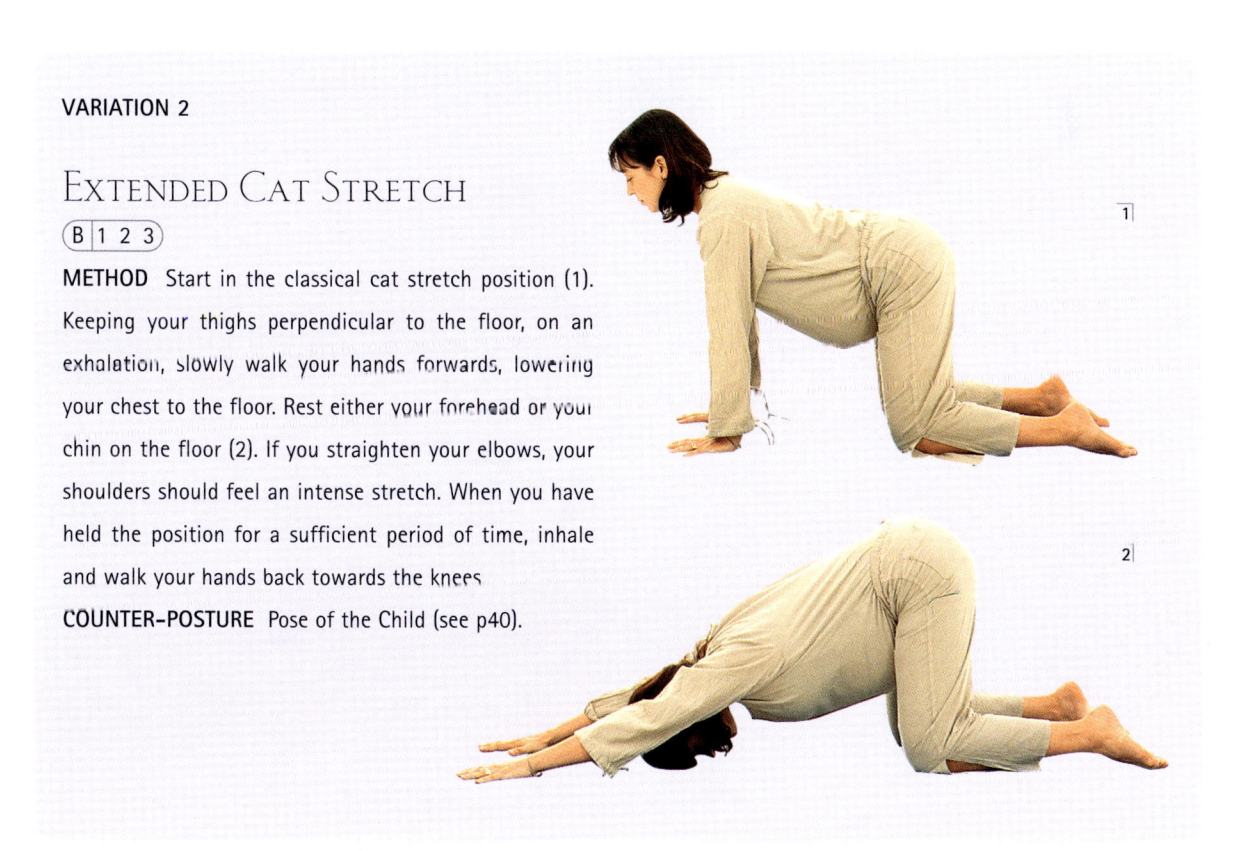

VARIATION 2

Extended Cat Stretch
(B | 1 2 3)

METHOD Start in the classical cat stretch position (1). Keeping your thighs perpendicular to the floor, on an exhalation, slowly walk your hands forwards, lowering your chest to the floor. Rest either your forehead or your chin on the floor (2). If you straighten your elbows, your shoulders should feel an intense stretch. When you have held the position for a sufficient period of time, inhale and walk your hands back towards the knees.
COUNTER-POSTURE Pose of the Child (see p40).

Sitting and Supine Postures

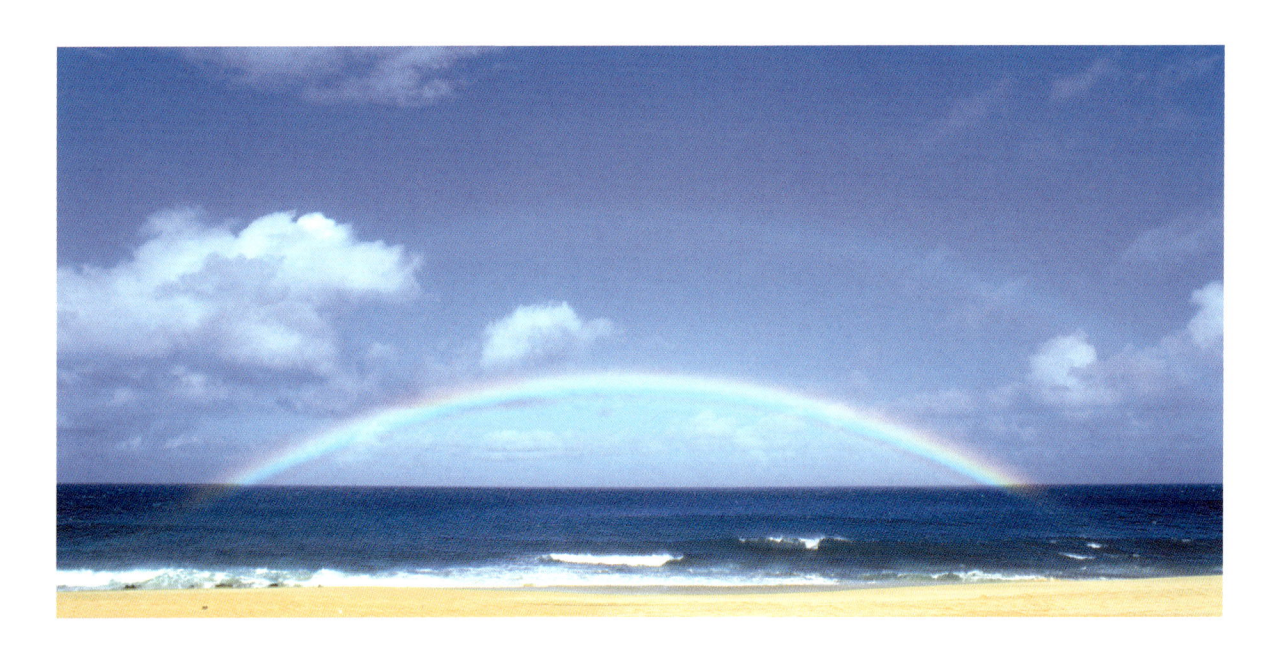

THE BRIDGE

Setu Bandhasana

B 1 2

BENEFITS Brings strength and flexibility to the spine.

CAUTIONS It is essential to keep the buttock muscles and the thighs firmly clenched for the duration of the exercise to protect the muscles in the lower back as the spine curves.

METHOD Lie flat on the floor with your legs bent. Draw your heels as close to your buttocks as possible, with your feet hip distance apart and parallel to each other. Let your arms lie alongside your body with your hands, palms down, next to your buttocks (1). Ensure that your chin is not pointing up towards the ceiling, as this compacts the vertebrae in the back of the neck. Tighten your buttock muscles and feel what happens. The pelvis lifts off the floor and the small of your back pushes down. Release your buttock muscles.

Take a preparatory breath, in and out. Inhale and tighten your buttocks, lifting your pelvis and slowly raising your hips towards the ceiling, gradually lifting your spine off the floor, one vertebra at a time, until your hips reach their peak (2).

Start exhaling and slowly lower your spine back down to the floor. Repeat the exercise six times. As you move, you should feel as if there is a wave passing through your spine.

COUNTER-POSTURE Apanasana (see p39).

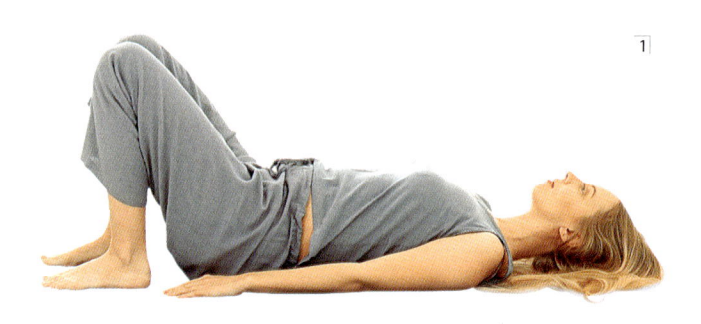

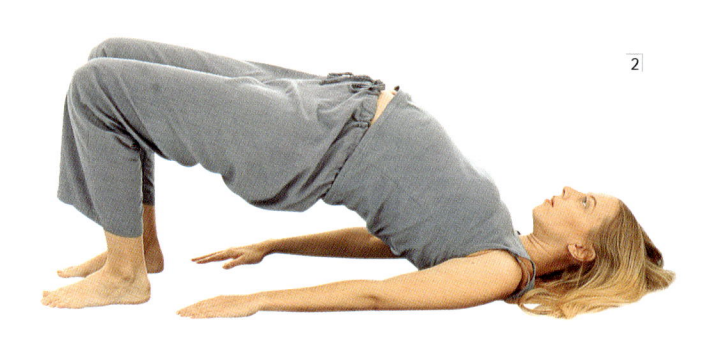

The Bridge

VARIATION 1

(1 | 2)

BENEFITS Stretches the spine and the hips.

The starting position for this variation is the same as for the main posture. This time, place your right ankle on top of your left knee, turning your right knee out and pushing it down towards the floor (1). Keeping your hands on the floor beside you, inhale and raise your hips slowly up towards the ceiling (2), then slowly lower them on the exhalation. Keep pushing your right knee down towards the floor while raising and lowering your hips. Do this exercise three more times and then change legs, placing your left ankle on your right knee. Repeat the exercise four times on the other side. This is an excellent hip stretch. Remember to keep the buttocks clenched.

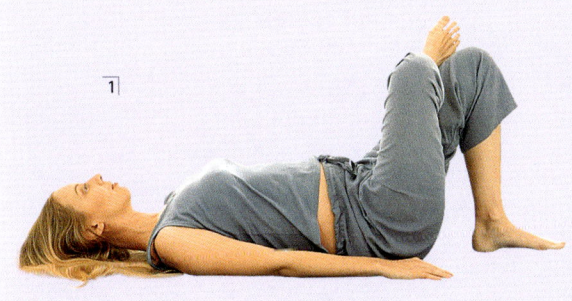

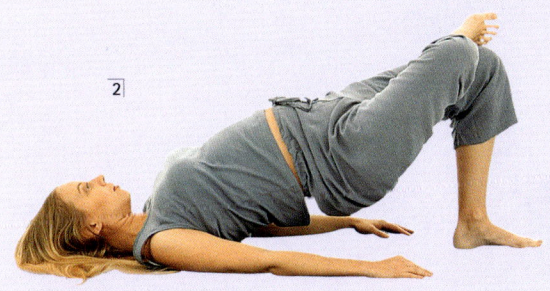

VARIATION 2

(1 | 2)

BENEFITS Releases tension in the lower spine.

The starting position is the same as for the main posture. Inhale, tighten your buttocks and raise your hips towards the ceiling (be careful not to overstretch your abdominal muscles). When your hips have reached their peak, hold them there and bend your elbows, placing your hands under your hips with your fingers pointing outwards (1). Make sure that you are not holding your breath. Carefully walk your feet away from you (2) until you can straighten them completely (3). Hold the posture for as long as it is comfortable. To come out of it, walk your feet back to their original position (1), then remove your hands and, on an exhalation, slowly lower your hips to the floor. Draw your knees onto your chest and hug them.

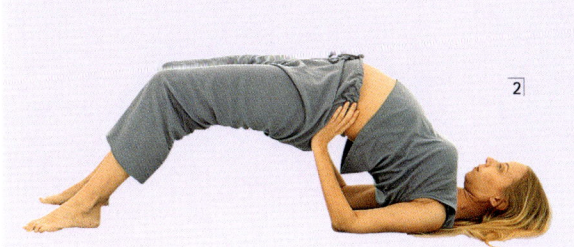

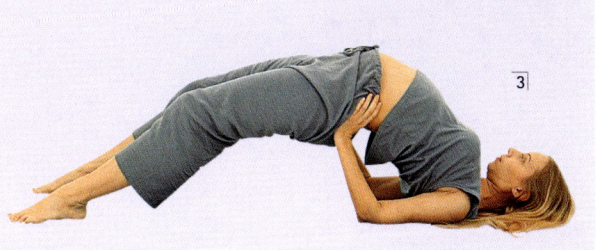

49

Sitting and Supine Postures

THE STAFF

(This posture is also called the Walking Stick.)

Dandasana

(B|1 2 3)

BENEFITS Strengthens the legs and the spine, and increases energy.

METHOD Sit on your mat with legs stretched out in front of you. Pull your toes up, push your knees down and stretch into your heels so firmly that they pop up off the floor (above). Stretch your arms away from you at a 45-degree angle and stretch firmly through the fingertips. Lift your sternum and relax your shoulders. Hold the position and practise the Ujjayi breath. You should feel a two-way movement of energy from your hips, down into your heels and up towards the crown of your head. Beware of this exercise. It looks innocuous, but you may find it so strenuous that you almost stop breathing.

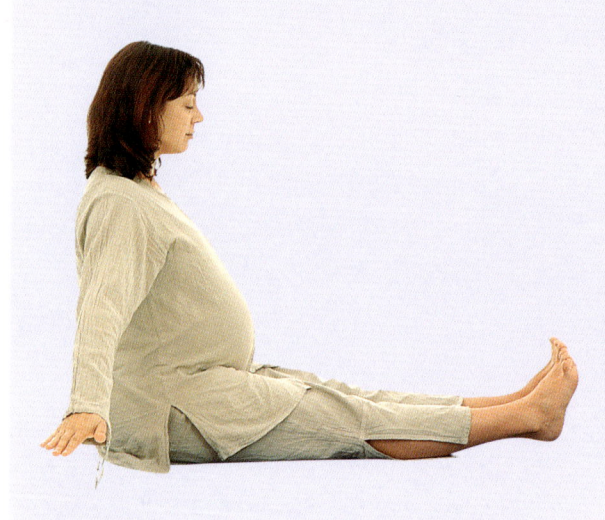

COUNTER-POSTURE Relax out of the posture and shake your legs.

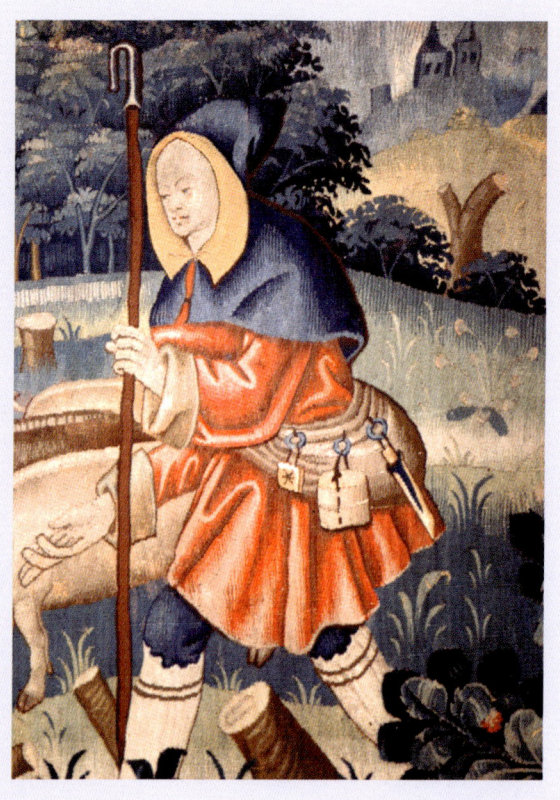

VARIATION

(I|1 2 3)

Start in the same position as for the main posture. Inhale and raise your right foot as high as possible. Keep your foot flexed and hold it up while you exhale and inhale, then lower it to the ground on the next exhalation. Repeat four times with each foot. This is a strenuous exercise that works the abdominal muscles, so stop if it feels uncomfortable.

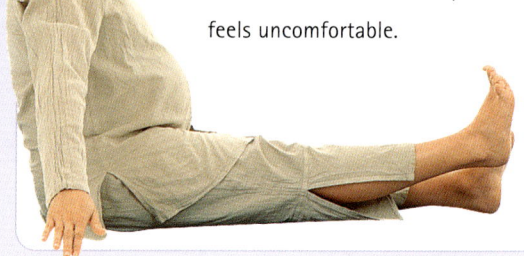

Head to Knee Posture

(This posture is also called the One Leg Forward Bend.)

Janu Sirsasana

(1 | 2)

CAUTIONS Do not bend the spine – keep it long and straight, folding from the hips. Only extend as far as is comfortable.

BENEFITS A calming pose that stretches the hamstrings, spine and hips. It aids digestion and relieves urinary problems.

METHOD Sit on your mat with your legs stretched out in front of you. Bend your left knee, drawing your heel into the perineum (groin) and trying to get the knee as close to the floor as possible. Push your right knee down towards the floor, pull up your toes and extend into your right heel (1). Place your finger-tips in your hip joints and gently rock backwards and forwards. The hip joint is like the hinge in a door and should work in the same manner (opening and closing). As you rock forwards, keep your spine erect. This is not the full posture; it is just to give you the feeling of the exercise.

To get into the full posture, inhale and slowly raise your arms sideways above your head (2). Exhale, stretch forward from your hips and reach for your outstretched foot, keeping your spine straight (3). If you cannot reach your foot without bending your spine, use a strap to assist you (see below). Hold the posture for as long as it is comfortable, keeping a regular, deep breathing rhythm, then inhale and raise your arms forwards above your head, before lowering them slowly sideways on the exhalation. Shake out your legs and repeat the exercise with the opposite leg. Remember to work both sides of the body equally and for the same period of time.

COUNTER-POSTURE Pose of the Child (see p40) or Apanasana (see p39).

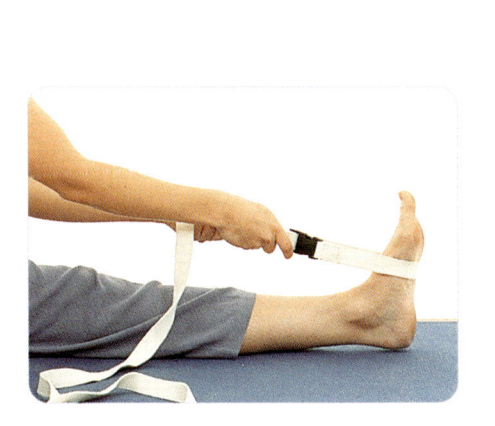

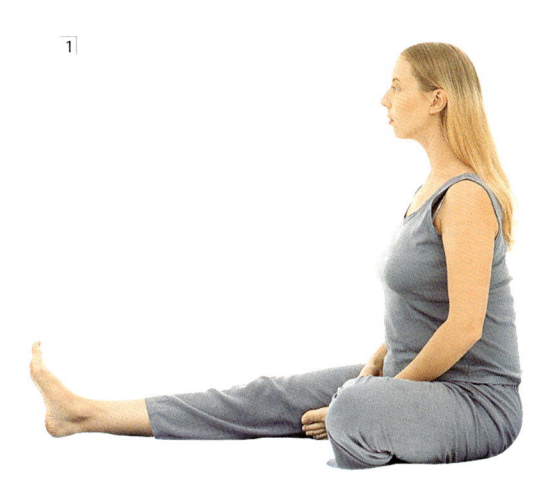

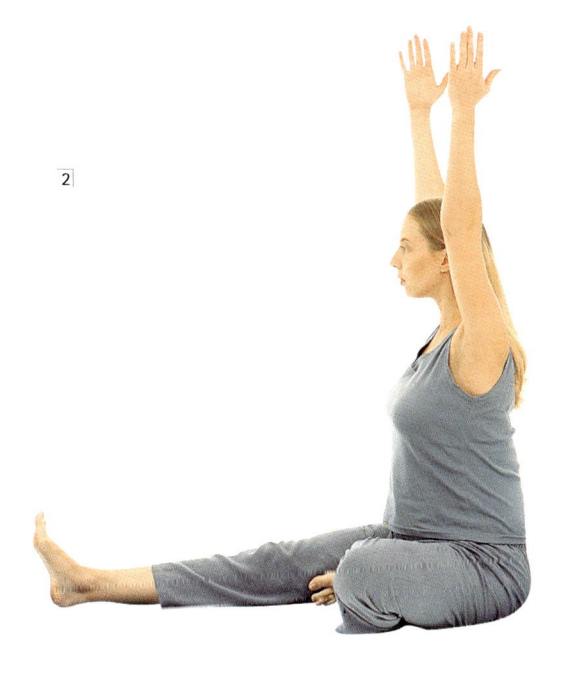

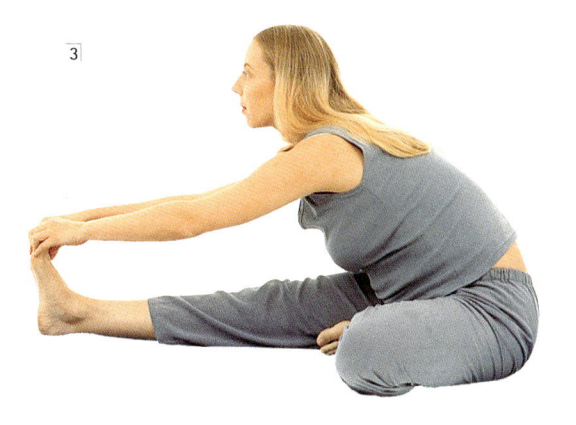

Sitting and Supine Postures

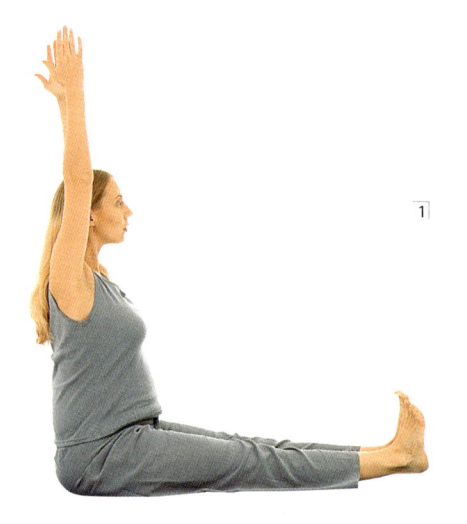

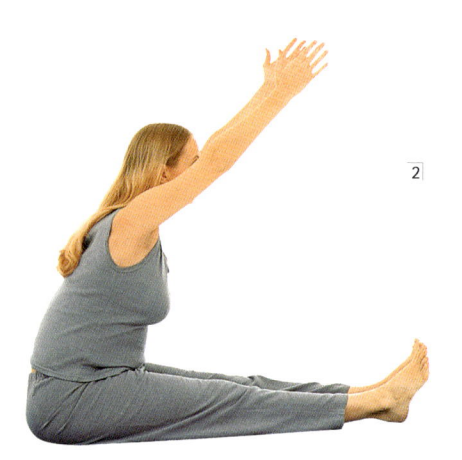

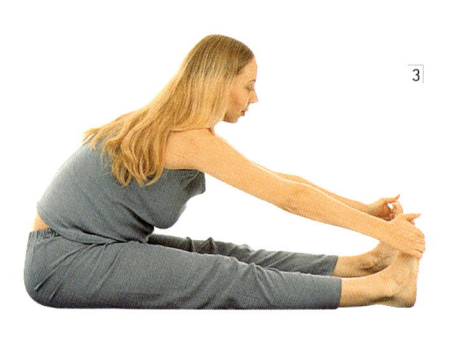

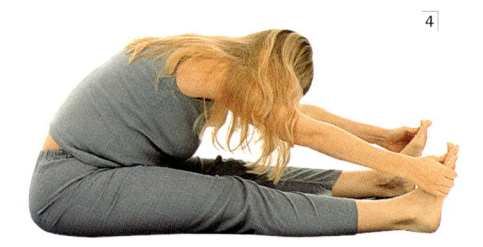

SITTING FORWARD BEND
Paschimottasana

(1 | 2 3)

BENEFITS Stretches the spine, hamstrings, Achilles tendon and hips. Massages the liver, pancreas and kidneys and aids peristaltic movement, thus improving digestion. It also has an exceptionally calming effect on the mind.

CAUTIONS Keep your spine erect. As your abdomen expands, it will be necessary do this exercise with your feet slightly apart.

METHOD Sit with your legs together and stretched out in front of you. Push both knees down towards the floor and stretch into your heels. Pull up your toes. Lift your sternum to lengthen your spine and relax your shoulders. Place your fingertips inside your hip joints and gently rock backwards and forwards to get the feeling of the posture. Inhale and stretch your arms, palms up, to the side and up above your head (1). On the exhalation stretch forwards from your hips (2), and take hold of your feet (3). Keep your spine in a straight line. If you cannot reach your feet, use a strap. Hold for as long as it is comfortable, breathing deeply. Now, relax into the position. Let your knees bend a little and allow your feet to soften. Drop your head down towards your knees and let your spine relax (4). Close your eyes and breathe deeply. When your body feels that it has had enough, inhale and stretch your arms forward, away from you and sweep them up above your head. On the exhalation stretch them down towards the floor.

COUNTER-POSTURE Pose of the Child (see p40) or Apanasana (see p39).

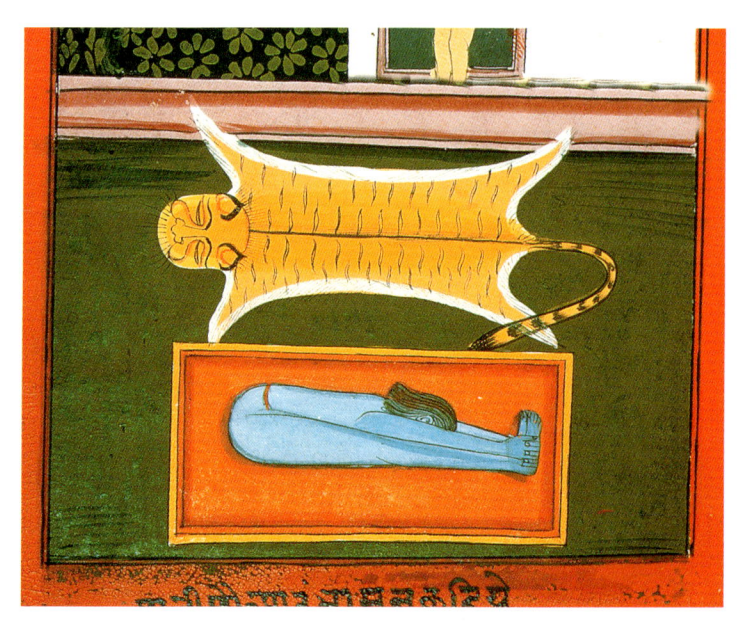

52

Open Leg Forward Bend

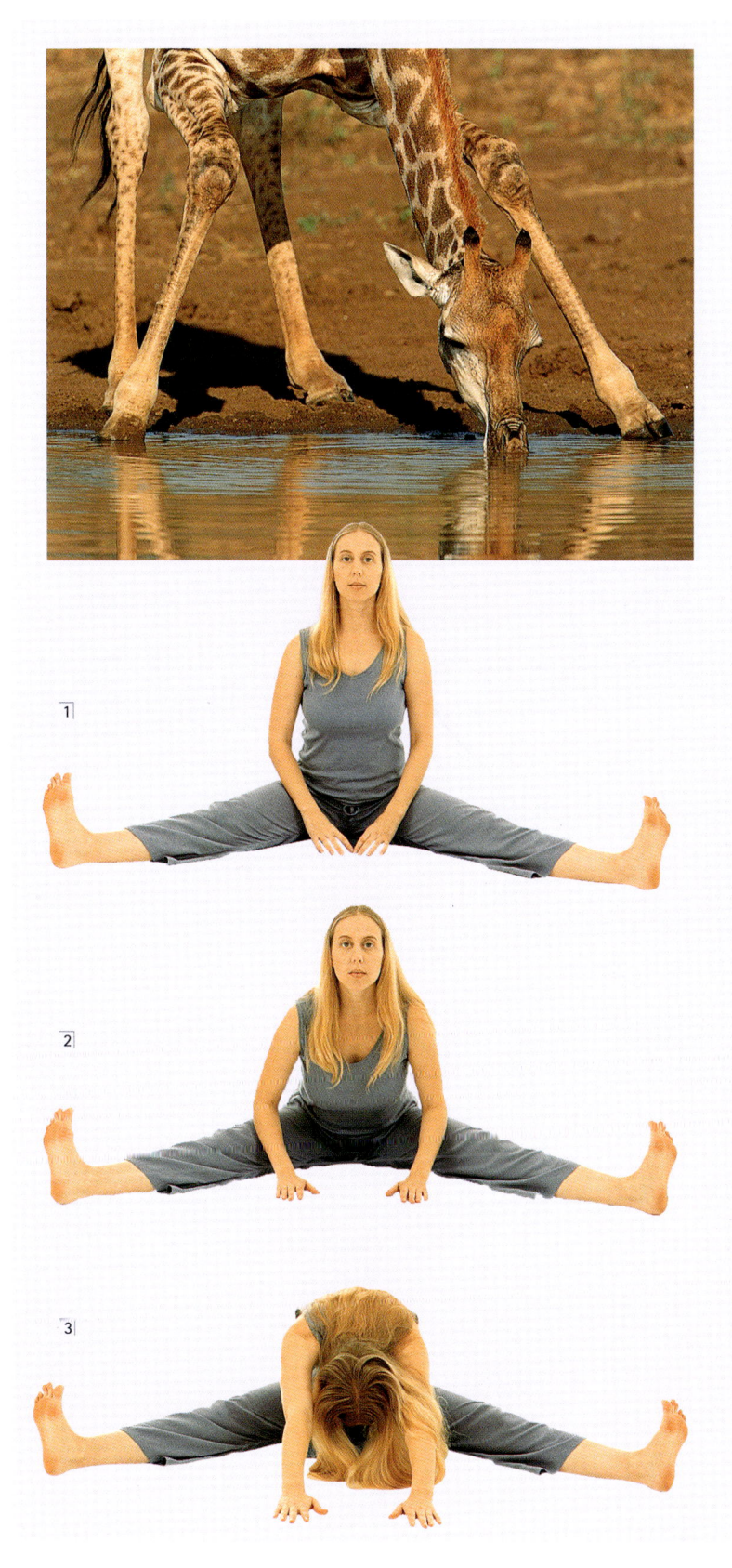

OPEN LEG FORWARD BEND
Upavistha Konasana

(1 | 2 3)

BENEFITS Stretches the inner thigh muscles and the spine, and opens the hips and pelvic area.

CAUTIONS Keep your spine straight. Don't drop your head below the level of your heart if you suffer from high blood pressure.

METHOD Sit on your mat with your legs open as wide as is comfortably possible. Stretch into your heels and pull up your toes (1). Place your hands on the floor in front of you. Keep your spine straight and gently rock backwards and forwards to get the feel of the posture (2). Exhale and walk your hands away from you, keeping your back flat and bringing your chest as close to the floor as possible (3). Do not round your back, as this will compress the abdominal area.

Hold the posture for a comfortable period, breathing deeply and evenly. Close your eyes and relax into the position. On an inhalation, walk your hands back towards you, raising your head and spine and coming into the natural sitting position. Bring your legs together and give them a shake.

COUNTER-POSTURE Apanasana (see p39).

Sitting and Supine Postures

Lunges and Leg Stretches moving into the Monkey God Posture (splits)

Hanumanasana

Beginners and intermediate students should concentrate on the lunges and stretches, leaving the splits to advanced practitioners. Do not stretch beyond your limits. The benefits and cautions below apply to all three exercises.

BENEFITS These postures stretch the quadriceps (front thigh muscle), hamstrings and hips. The lunges and stretches should be performed with a flowing rhythm.
CAUTIONS It is essential that your ankle is directly under your knee during the lunges and leg stretches. If your foot is not correctly positioned, you could damage your knee. Kneeling on a blanket will help to protect your knees.

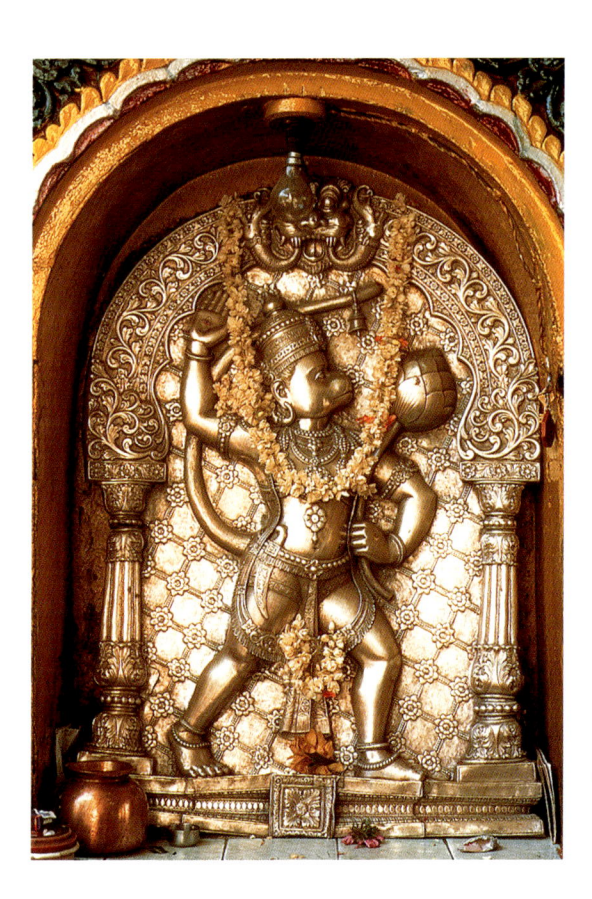

Lunges

B | 1 | 2 | 3

METHOD Sit on your knees and raise your buttocks so that you are in an upright kneeling position (1). Take a large step forwards with your right foot. Inhale, and as you exhale, lunge forwards, sinking into your left hip. Drop your groin as close to the floor as possible, keeping your right knee above your ankle (2). Rock gently back and forwards, or hold the position for six Ujjayi breaths.

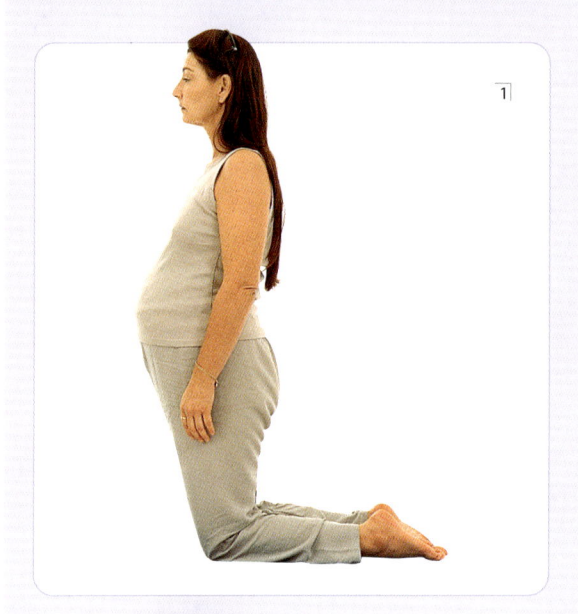

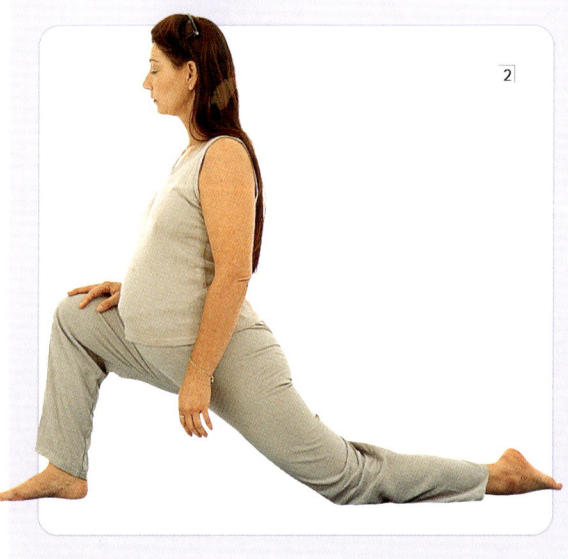

Lunges and Leg Stretches

LEG STRETCHES
1 | 2 3

CAUTIONS Do not over-flex your back knee.

METHOD Continuing from the previous position, lift your left foot off the floor, hold it in your left hand and draw it up towards your buttocks (1). Increase the lunge into your left hip. If necessary, place your right hand on the floor for balance. When the thigh muscles have been sufficiently stretched, release your left foot and place it back on the floor. Take a recovery breath, in and out.

Inhale and as you exhale, rock back, straighten your right leg, pull up your toes and slide your right heel 2cm (1in) forward along the floor (2). Balance yourself with your hands and inhale. As you exhale, move your buttocks slightly backwards and stretch your head and torso out over your right leg. Be gentle, this is a big stretch. Do not bend your right knee. Hold the position for as long as it is comfortable, then raise your head and torso back to an upright position on an inhalation.

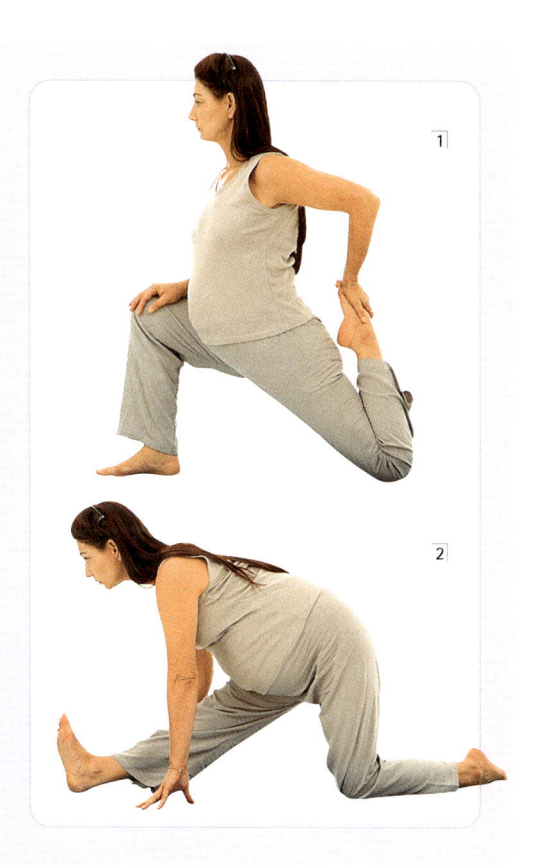

SPLITS (HANUMANASANA)
A | 1 2 3

CAUTIONS This is a posture for advanced practitioners. Do not attempt it unless your hamstrings are flexible and supple and you are thoroughly warmed up beforehand.

METHOD Start from posture 2 above (with your right leg stretched out in front of you). Relax and take a recovery breath. Supporting yourself on your hands, exhale and slowly slide your right leg forward as far as comfortable, simultaneously straightening your left leg. If you can, take the weight off your hands and bring them into the prayer position. Do not hold this posture for too long as it is strenuous. To come out of the splits, take your weight onto your hands again.

Inhale, and draw your right leg back, bending your left leg to return to a kneeling position. Relax, then repeat the exercise with the left leg in front.

COUNTER-POSTURE Sit with your legs stretched out in front of you and shake them slowly from side to side to release built-up tension. Rest in the Pose of the Child.

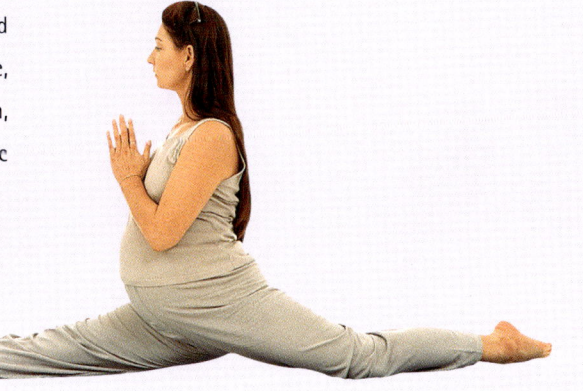

Sitting and Supine Postures

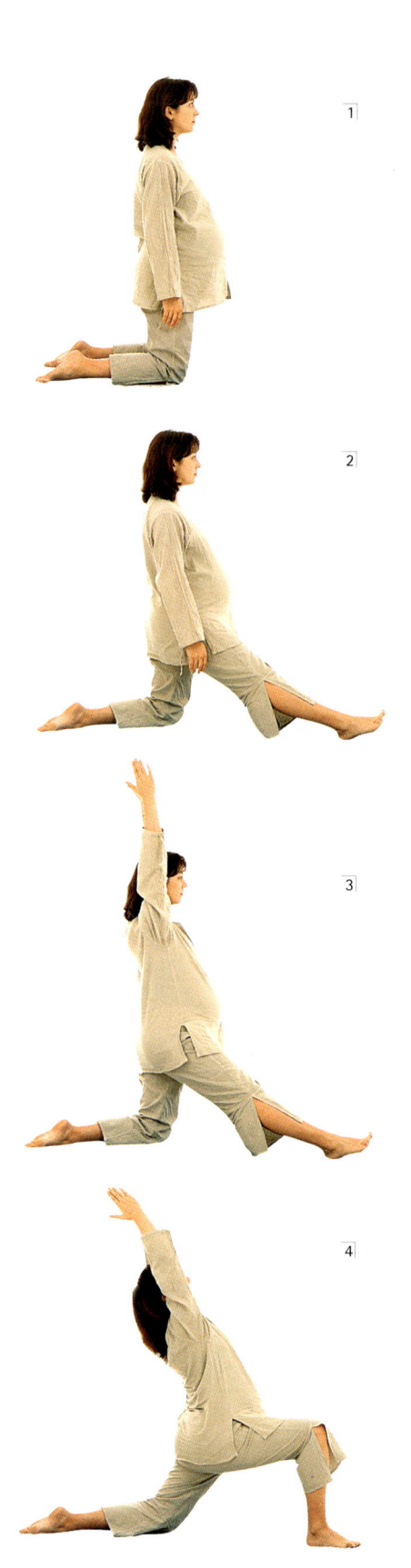

THE CRESCENT MOON

Chandrasana

(1 2 3)

BENEFITS This stimulating posture opens the hips and brings about flexibility of the spine. It also opens the chest and heart area, and stimulates the kidneys and the adrenal glands.

CAUTIONS Do not drop your head back if you suffer from neck problems. If you have high blood pressure, do not take your hands above your head. Rather place them in the prayer position in front of your sternum. The ankle should be directly underneath the knee during this posture. It might be necessary to kneel on a blanket to protect your knees. Take care not to overstretch in this posture.

METHOD Sit on your knees and raise your buttocks so that you are in a full kneeling position (1). Inhale and as you exhale stretch your right leg straight out in front of you (2). On your next inhalation bring your arms forwards and away from you, lifting them above your head (3). If you suffer from high blood pressure, rather place your hands in the prayer position on the sternum (below). As you exhale, bend your right knee so that you are in a lunging position, sinking into your left hip and stretching upwards (4). Try to straighten your elbows, but keep the shoulders soft. Ensure that your right ankle is directly under your knee. If you don't have a neck problem, gently drop your head back to look up at your hands. If you have a supple back, then lean slightly backwards.

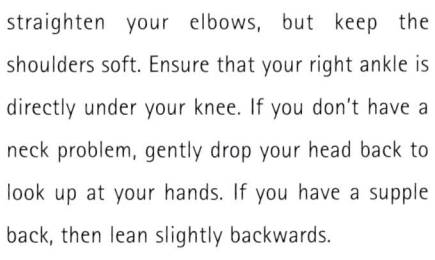

Hold the posture for as long as it feels comfortable. To come out of it, inhale and look forward as you rock back gently onto your left leg, straightening your right leg. As you exhale, lower your arms sideways and down. Keep the arms strong and do not bend your elbows. Draw your right leg underneath you into a kneeling position. Relax in the Pose of the Child before repeating the posture with the left leg in front. This is a truly elegant-looking posture. It is, however, quite strong.

COUNTER-POSTURE The Pose of the Child (see p40) or Apanasana (see p39).

56

The Fish

Matsyasana

(1 | 2)

BENEFITS Opens and expands the throat and chest, and strengthens the upper back and spine. Increases blood flow to the head, stimulating the pituitary and pineal glands, and the thyroid and parathyroid glands in the throat. It encourages deep breathing, so is beneficial to asthma sufferers. It also alleviates piles.

CAUTIONS This posture can be uncomfortable if you suffer from neck and knee problems. If you do not enjoy it, then leave it out.

METHOD The Fish is traditionally done in the Lotus position (see p43), but a variation is provided for those who have not yet mastered this posture. Start by sitting in the Lotus position (1) and lean back, resting your weight on your elbows (2). Raise your sternum (chest) towards the ceiling and gently drop your head backwards. As your head comes closer to the floor bring your elbows in towards your buttocks (3). When the crown of your head is resting on the floor, release the weight from your elbows and take hold of your big toes with your hands (4). To come out of the pose, take your weight back onto your elbows and place your hands on the floor. Straighten your arms, lifting yourself up into a sitting position. This posture is not nearly as complex or difficult as it looks. If you practise it in a swimming pool, you will float lightly on the surface of the water.

COUNTER-POSTURE Apanasana (see p39).

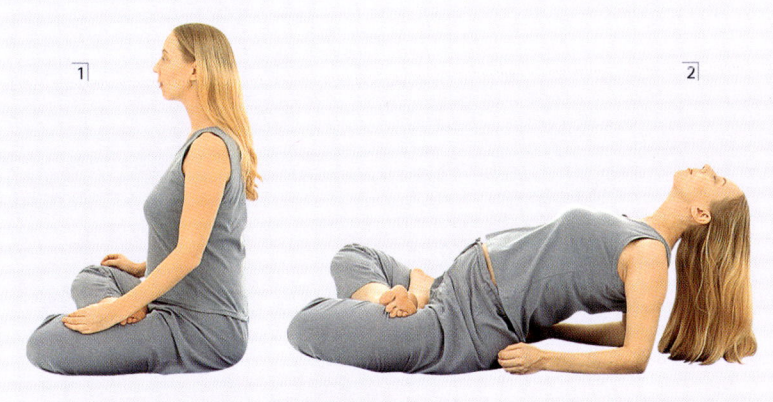

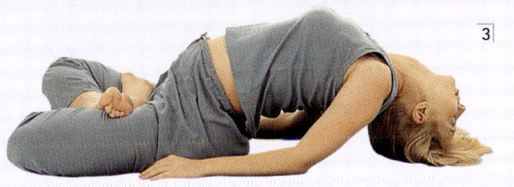

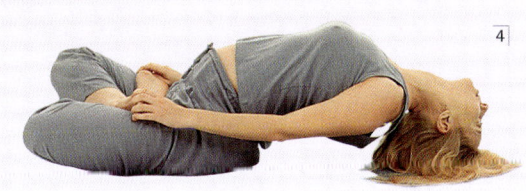

VARIATION

(1 | 2)

CAUTIONS Don't attempt this if you suffer from knee problems.

METHOD Start by sitting on your knees. Lean backwards and place your elbows on the floor. Gently drop your head and slide your elbows towards your buttocks. When the crown of your head touches the floor, place your hands on your chest in the prayer position. Then, keeping your hands together, take your arms over your head to the floor behind you.

If the stretch in your quadriceps (thigh muscles) is too intense, open your knees slightly.

COUNTER-POSTURE Apanasana (see p39).

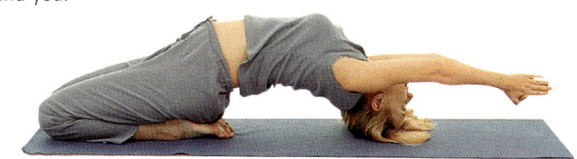

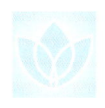

STANDING *postures refresh the body and mind by removing tension and physical stress. They teach the principles of correct movement and develop strength, stability and balance, all of which are essential to our daily lives, regardless of whether we are walking, sitting or standing. Standing postures benefit the back, neck, spine and shoulders. They strengthen the legs, enabling them to carry the additional weight of the growing foetus. When you work in these postures, circulation and breathing improve, aches and pains are relieved, and digestion is stimulated.*

As your pregnancy progresses, your centre of gravity will shift and you may find that you start to lean forwards. Yoga helps to centre you, aligning your body and improving your posture.

It is important to work on a flat, level surface and to make quite sure that you can't slip or fall. It is normal to jump into many standing postures, but this is not advised during pregnancy, and you should rather step or walk into them. If you suffer from high blood pressure or a heart condition, remember not to raise your hands above your head, or lower your head below the level of your heart.

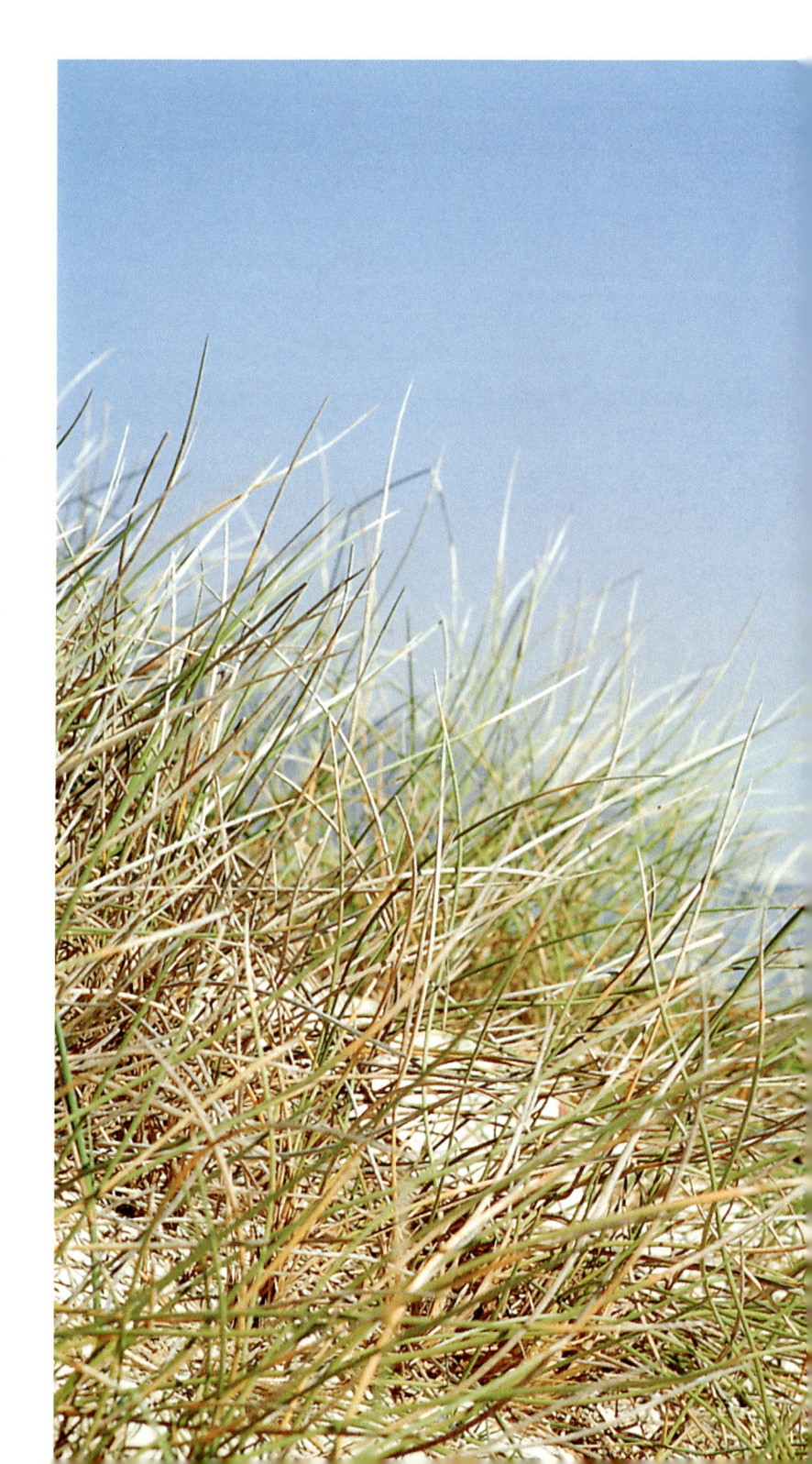

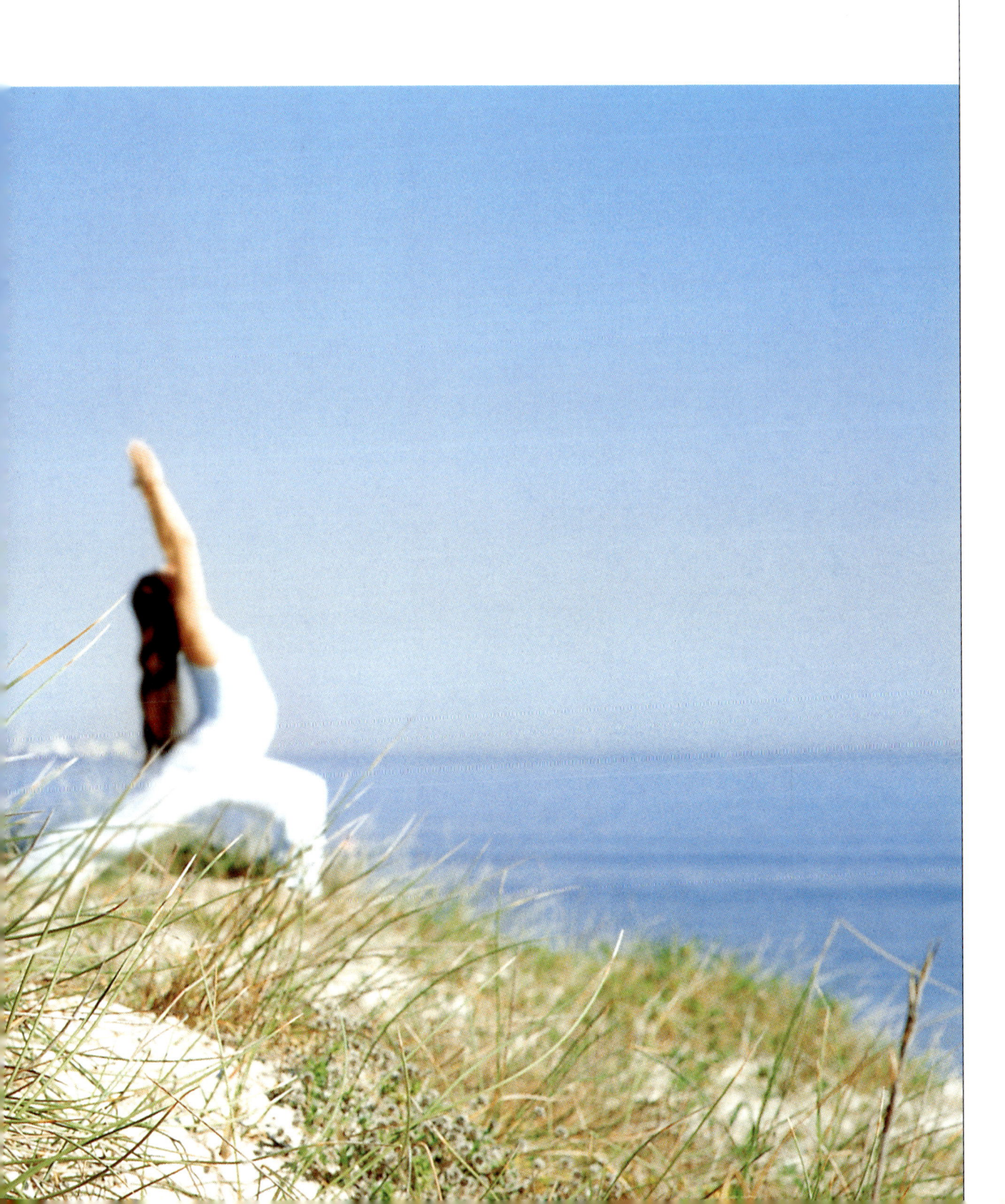

Standing Postures

Standing Postures

Upright Standing posture
Samasthiti

In Sanksrit, *sama* means 'equal' and *sthiti* means 'stay' or 'balance'. Thus *Samasthiti* implies 'being at one with yourself', or bringing the body into balance and harmony with the intellect, the emotions and the breath.

B | 1 2 3

BENEFITS This posture is calming and 'grounding'. It is used as a rest posture after practising strenuous standing poses.

METHOD Stand with your feet hip distance apart and parallel to each other. Make sure that your weight is evenly distributed on both feet. Close your eyes and keep them closed for the duration of this posture. Relax your knees (do not bend them, just ensure that the kneecaps are not pulled back and locked). Check that you are not clenching your teeth and that your tongue is lying softly in the base of your mouth, not stuck to your palate. Relax your shoulders. Feel the space between your ear lobes and your shoulders, as if your shoulders were falling softly down away from your ears.

In your mind's eye, follow that softness down your arms, through your hands, past your wrists and down into your fingertips and feel it moving down your spine. Relax first your stomach muscles and then your buttock muscles. Follow the softness down your legs, past your knees and into your feet. Imagine your feet are growing roots into the earth. Feel any discomfort or distress from the day moving away from your brain, travelling down your spine and legs and out of the soles of your feet. The longer you hold this posture, the more calming it will be. This is an excellent posture with which to start your yoga session. Your breathing should remain calm and steady throughout.

The Mountain
Tadasana

B | 1 2 3

BENEFITS This is a rejuvenating and energizing posture. It also improves balance and steadiness.

METHOD Stand with your feet together, with the big toes, heels and ankles touching each other. (As your abdomen expands you may need to keep your feet hip width apart). Close your eyes and keep them closed for the duration of the posture. Draw your inner thigh muscles firmly together. You will feel your buttocks become energized. Tighten your buttock muscles a little more, continuing to draw the inner thigh muscles together. From the waist down to your feet you should feel as solid as a mountain, and from the waist up to the crown of your head you should feel as light as the clouds on top of the mountain. Your body might sway a little from side to side or backwards and forwards, but this is normal, as it is looking for its balance. Picture yourself growing roots out of the soles of your feet and feel as if you are pulling rejuvenating energy out of the earth, through your feet, up your legs, up your spine and into your head. When you feel that you have held the posture for a sufficient length of time, open your eyes and give your feet a shake.

It is a natural sequence to do the Mountain Posture immediately after Samasthiti. Move from the one posture into the other without opening your eyes.

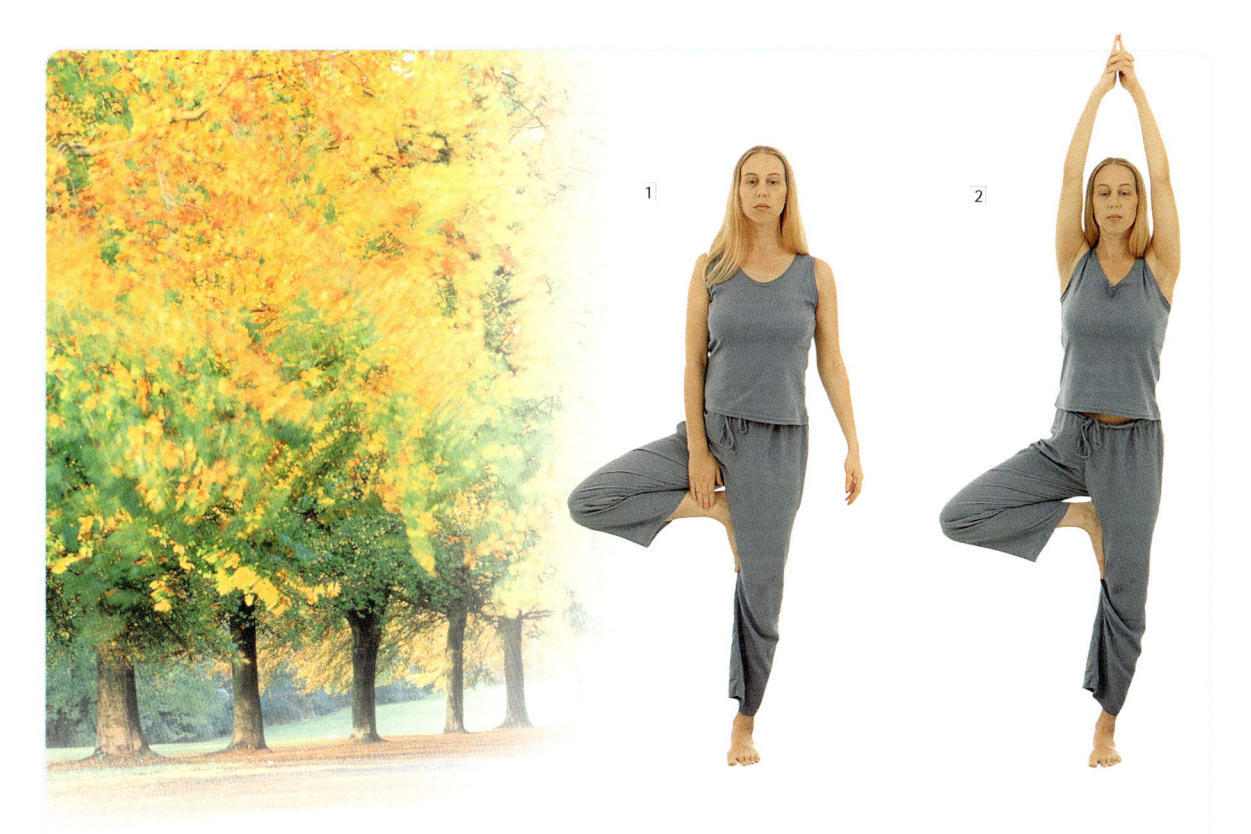

The Tree

Vrksasana

(B 1 2 3)

BENEFITS Improves balance and self-confidence, enhances concentration, strengthens the legs and opens the hips and pelvic area.

CAUTION Don't take your hands above your head if you suffer from high blood pressure.

METHOD Stand with your feet together and fix your eyes on a spot on the floor in front of you (this helps with concentration and stops you from falling over). You can also do this posture against a wall. Lift your right foot and place it as high up against the inner left thigh as possible, using your hand to guide your foot into position (1). Get your balance. Press your right foot firmly into the thigh to stop it from slipping down. Once you feel comfortable standing on one leg, draw your right knee as far back as it will go. This opens and stretches the hip and groin area.

Inhale and slowly raise your arms sideways above your head (2), or place them in the prayer position (3). Hold the posture for as long as possible. Exhale, lowering your arms sideways, and place your right foot back on the ground. Take a recovery breath and repeat with the left foot against the right thigh.

Sometimes you can concentrate so intensely on trying to balance that you forget to breathe. If you concentrate on breathing, the body will automatically balance. If you are holding your breath you will fall over.

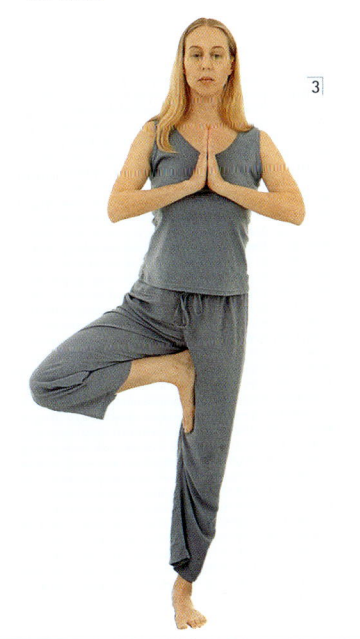

Standing Postures

The Dancer
Natarajasana

[1 | 2 3]

BENEFITS Improves balance, opens up the hips and stretches the quadriceps (thigh muscles). Enhances self-confidence and concentration.

CAUTION Take care that you are properly balanced. Use a chair or a partner for support until you are confident enough to do it alone.

METHOD Stand with both feet together. Fix your eyes on a spot on the floor in front of you. Raise the right foot behind you and take hold of it with your right hand (1). Draw the heel as close as possible towards the right buttock, keeping both knees in line (this is called the foot lift). Hold the posture for six breaths while you stretch the quadriceps (the large muscles at the front of the thigh). The closer the foot comes to the buttocks, the bigger the stretch in the thigh. Inhale, and raise your left hand up towards the ceiling, then stretch your right foot away from the buttocks and curve it up behind you (2), moving into the Dancer. Hold the posture for as long as it is comfortable. Release your foot and place it back on the floor as you lower your left arm. Take a recovery breath and then repeat on the other side. Use a chair to help you balance when you are learning.

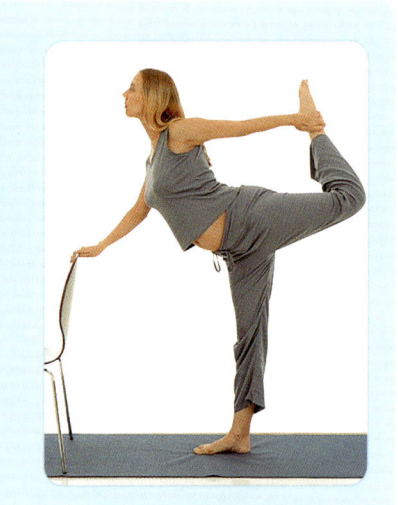

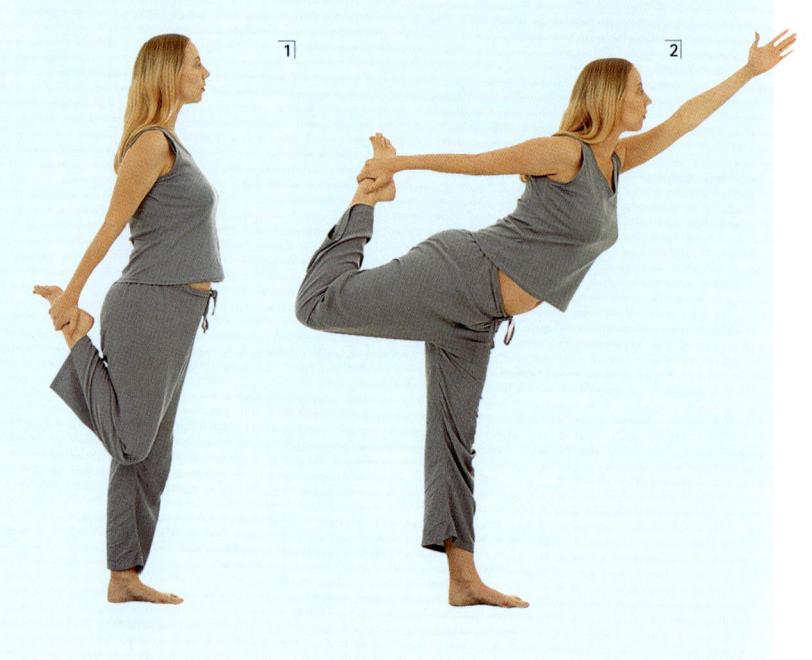

The Warrior (1)
Virabhadrasana No.1

[1 | 2 3]

BENEFITS Strengthens the entire body, especially the quadriceps, and increases the heartbeat.

CAUTIONS Neck, high blood pressure, lower back. Do not raise your hands above your head if you suffer from high blood pressure. When you lunge forward, make sure that bent knee remains directly in line with the ankle; if you over- or underextend your knee you could damage it. If you suffer from lower back problems then do not lean backwards in this posture, keep the body upright instead. If you have a neck problem, it is better to keep looking straight ahead than upwards. This is a strenuous posture.

METHOD Stand with your feet as far apart as possible and parallel to each other (1). Turn your right foot out at a 90-degree angle and turn the toes of your left foot inwards at a 45-degree angle. The heel of the right foot must be in line

The Warrior

with the instep of the left foot. Turn towards your right and place your hands on your hips (2). Move your right hip back as far as it will go and bring your left hip forwards, bringing the tops of the inner thighs together. Make sure your weight is even on both feet. Look straight ahead.

Inhale and stretch your arms sideways, with the palms facing upwards, above your head to end with the palms facing each other. Straighten your arms and relax your shoulders (3). Alternatively, place your hands in front of your chest, in the prayer position.

As you exhale, lunge with your right knee to form a right angle with the floor, bringing your groin as close to the floor as possible, and keeping the left leg straight behind you (4). Do not stop breathing. Check that your right knee is directly above your ankle. If not, then move your right foot to align it. Do not allow the right knee to collapse inwards. Gently drop your head and lean backwards as you look up at your hands. Try to keep your left heel on the ground. Hold the posture for as long as you can, keeping your breathing even and rhythmical.

To come out of the posture, inhale as you straighten your right knee and raise your head to look forward again. Exhale and slowly lower your arms sideways. Inhale and turn to the front, moving your feet so that they are parallel to each other. Drop into a floppy forward bend to rest. Inhale and come up slowly, bringing your head up last. Repeat on the left side.

COUNTER-POSTURE

Samasthiti (see p60), or relax in a floppy forward bend.

Standing Postures

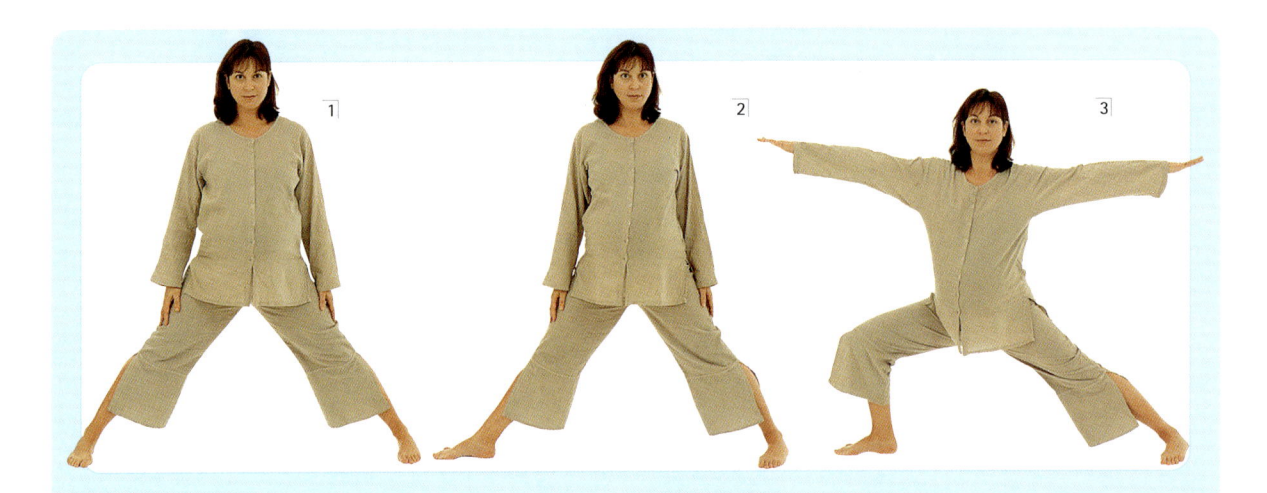

The Warrior (2)

Virabhadrasana No.2

BENEFITS Strengthens the entire body, especially the quadriceps, and increases the heartbeat.

CAUTIONS The ankle must be situated directly under the knee when you lunge. This is a strenuous posture, so do not hold it for longer than is comfortable. If you suffer from high blood pressure, keep your hands on your hips.

METHOD Stand with your feet as far apart as possible (1). Turn your right foot out at a 90-degree angle. Turn the toes of your left foot in at a 45-degree angle, ensuring that the right heel is in line with the left instep (2). Your hips should face forwards and should be level and even.

Inhale and raise your arms slowly sideways to shoulder height, with the palms facing downwards. Exhale and relax your shoulders as you stretch into the fingertips.

Inhale and, as you exhale, lunge with the right knee, bringing your groin as close to the floor as possible (3). Check that the right ankle is situated directly under the knee. If it is not, then move your right foot. Do not let the right knee collapse inwards. Bring your torso into a position that is perfectly perpendicular to the floor. Turn your head to look across your right hand. Hold the position for as long as it is comfortable while ensuring that your breathing is regular and even.

To come out of the position, inhale and straighten your right knee. Bring your head to the front. On the exhalation, lower your arms slowly to your sides. Bring your feet parallel to each other and drop down into a floppy forward bend to rest. Come up slowly on an inhalation, bringing your head up last. Repeat on the left.

COUNTER-POSTURE Samasthiti (see p60) or drop into a floppy forward bend.

Standing Forward Bend

Uttanasana or *Padahastasana*

BENEFITS Stretches the hips and the hamstrings, massages the internal organs and has a calming effect on the mind. The variation also stretches the shoulders.

CAUTION If you suffer from high blood pressure or any condition where your head should not be below your heart, then bend only halfway. As your pregnancy progresses, you may need to have your legs and feet a little apart. Bend only as far as your expanding abdomen allows you to.

Standing Forward Bend

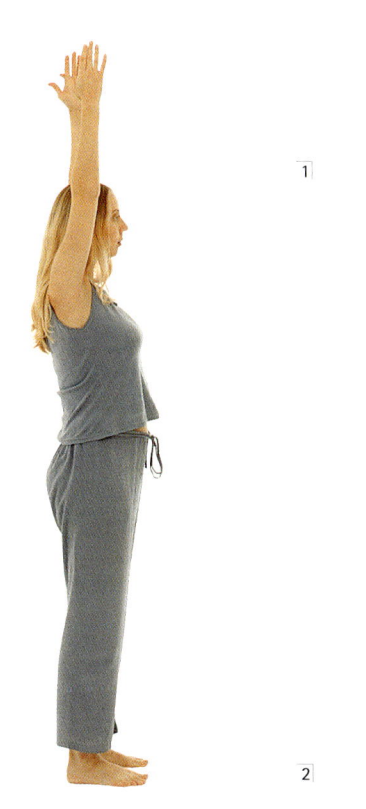

METHOD Stand with your legs and feet firmly together. Pull your kneecaps back and lock them. Inhale, extend your hands in front of you and raise them above your head (1). As you exhale, bend forward from the hips, stretch your arms away from you (2) and reach down towards your feet (3), all in a single flowing movement. (You can rest your hands on a chair or against a wall instead of bending all the way forward.) Ensure that you stretch forwards and out and try to keep your spine straight. Do not pull your shoulders up underneath your ears as you stretch forwards. Imagine that you are holding a ball between your outstretched hands, then placing it on the floor and rolling it towards your feet.

To come out of the posture, imagine that you are rolling the ball away from you, then lifting it up above your head on an inhalation. As you exhale, stretch your arms sideways and lower them to rest against the side of your body. Repeat the exercise six times. The last time you bend forward, try to hold the posture for six breaths.

Try not to bend your knees. It is better to keep them straight and hold your ankles or shins if you can't reach your toes. As your pregnancy advances and your abdomen expands, it may become necessary to have your feet a little apart to accommodate your belly.

COUNTER-POSTURE Shake your legs to release any tension that might have built up and then rest in Samasthiti (see p60).

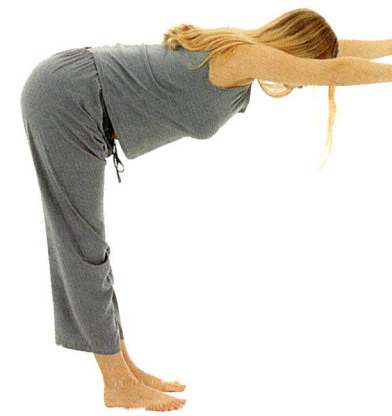

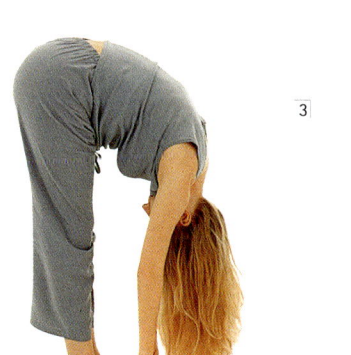

VARIATION

Padahastasana

Interlace your fingers behind your back. Inhale and lift your sternum, moving your hands as far away from your buttocks as possible (1). Exhale and stretch forwards, leading with your breastbone and bringing your chest down to your thighs. Lower your head and take your hands as far over your head as you can (2), resting your weight against a wall or chair if necessary. Hold the posture for as long as it feels comfortable.

To come up, inhale, raise your head and draw your arms towards your buttocks. Lift your chest and return to an upright position with a straight back. Exhale and shake your shoulders.

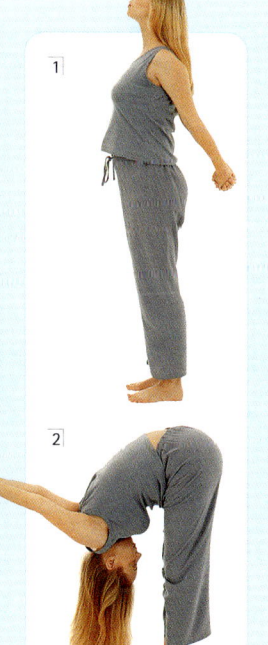

Standing Postures

SQUATS
Utkatasana

B | 1 2 3

BENEFITS This is an important exercise for pregnant women as it opens up the pelvic area and hips. It also strengthens the quadriceps.

CAUTION Use a chair for balance until you feel comfortable.

METHOD Stand with your feet hip distance apart and parallel to each other, turning the toes out slightly if necessary. (If your hips are not very supple, then place your feet a little further apart than hip distance.) Inhale and raise your arms in front of you to shoulder height, with the palms facing downwards (1). As you exhale, bend your knees and squat, bringing your buttocks as close to the floor as possible (2). Try to keep your knees as wide apart as you can.

If your heels lift off the floor, place wooden blocks, books or a telephone directory beneath them (see below). On an inhalation, tighten your quadriceps (thigh muscles) and raise yourself to a standing position using only the thigh muscles. Try not to push too hard against the floor with your feet; this may make it easier to stand up, but it does not strengthen the quadriceps. On the exhalation squat again.

Repeat this exercise three or four times. On the last squat, stay down and bring your hands into the prayer position. Put your elbows between your knees and use them to open your knees as wide as you can (3).

Hold the final position for as long as it is comfortable. To come up, release your hands, tighten your thigh muscles and use them to lift yourself up slowly.

COUNTER-POSTURE Shake your legs to release any tension that might have built up.

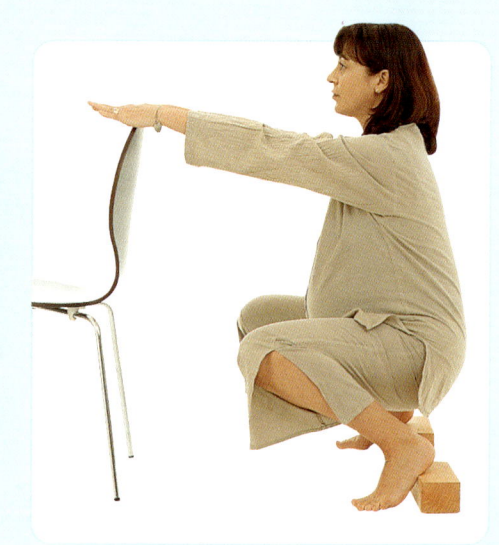

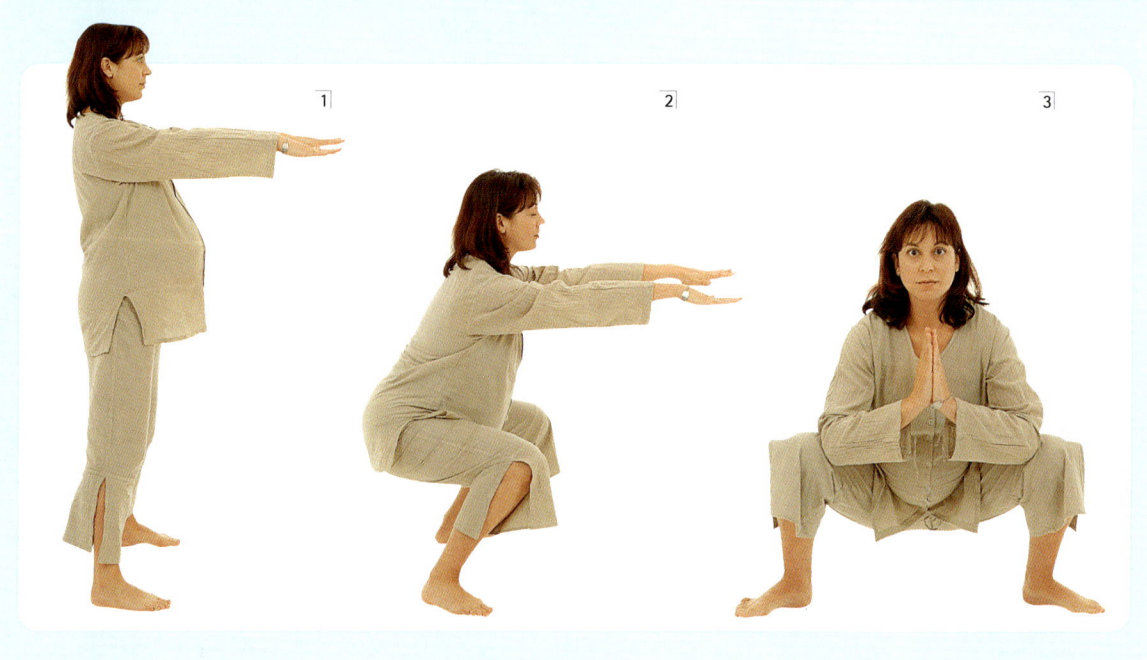

66

EXTENDED TRIANGLE POSTURE

Trikonasana

1 | 2 3

BENEFITS Increases lateral movement in the spine, strengthens the spine and legs, and massages the abdominal organs.

CAUTION This is a strenuous posture. Initially, you might like to practise with your back against a wall until you get the feeling of it and feel secure enough to do it without support.

METHOD Stand with your feet approximately 1m (3ft) apart and parallel to each other (1). Turn your right foot out at a 90-degree angle and bring the toes of your left foot in at a 45-degree angle. The heel of your right foot should be in line with your left instep. Ensure that your hips are facing forward and that they are level and even. Pull your kneecaps up. Push your weight into the outer aspect of your left foot (this is the foundation of the posture and will stop you from falling over). Inhale and raise your arms sideways to shoulder height, so that they are parallel to the floor. Let your palms face downwards (2). Exhale and relax your shoulders as you stretch into your fingertips. Inhale. As you exhale, extend from your hips over to the right as far as you can and then tilt downwards. Lightly rest your right hand on your right shin or on the floor. Take your left hand up vertically towards the ceiling with the palm facing forwards. Look up at the palm of your left hand (3). If you experience tension in the neck area, look forward or down. Keep pushing into the outer aspect of the left foot and keep your kneecaps pulled up. Breathe regularly and evenly and hold the posture for as long as it is comfortable. While doing this pose, you should imagine that there is a wall behind you and that your hips, shoulders, arms and head are flat against the wall.

To come out of the posture, inhale and feel as though you are being pulled up by your left hand, bringing the arms parallel to the floor. Lower the arms to the side of the body on the exhalation. Bring your feet parallel to each other again and drop into a floppy forward bend to rest. When you feel rested, inhale and come up slowly with a round back, bringing your head up last. Bring your feet together and give them a shake. Now do the entire posture with the left side of your body.

COUNTER-POSTURE Samasthiti (see p60) or relax in a floppy forward bend.

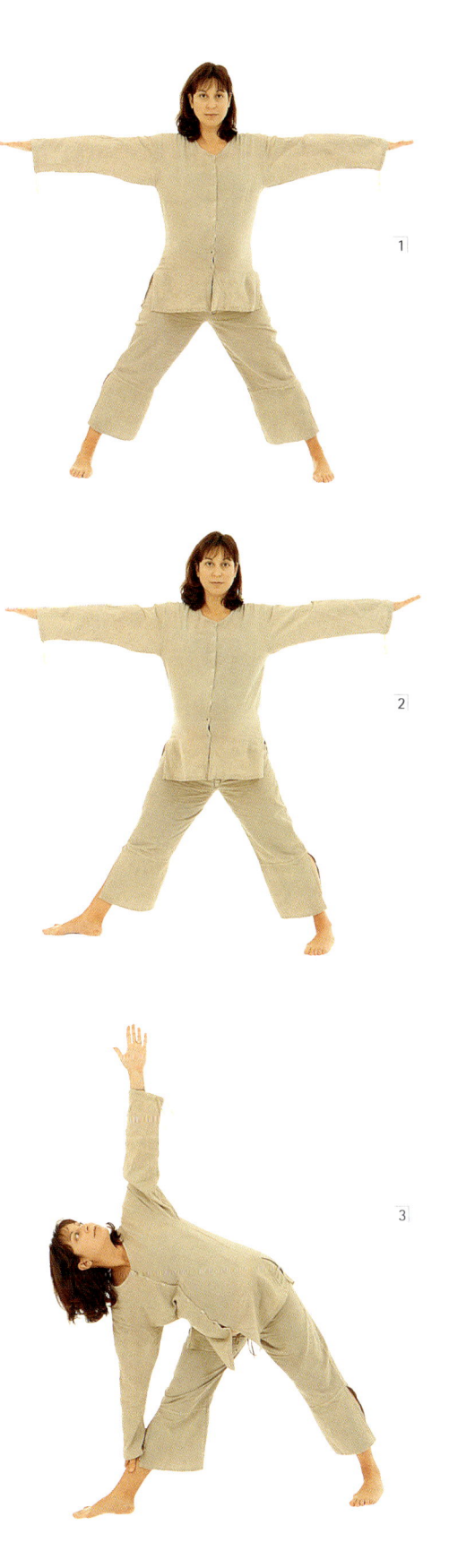

Standing Postures

Salute to the Sun
Surya Namaskar

1 | 2 3

BENEFITS This sequence of 12 postures which flow into each other is one of the most important in yoga. It works almost every muscle in the body and has a definite cardiovascular effect, so it is essential to get the breathing rhythm correct. If you do not have time to do a full yoga session every day, try to do five or six rounds of Salute to the Sun, followed by a period of relaxation and breathing, accompanied by quiet, gentle music.

CAUTIONS As your abdomen expands it will become necessary to do this sequence with the feet hip distance apart. Postures 6 (the Caterpillar) and 7 (the Cobra) will also have to be left out. In other words, you will move directly from the Plank into the Downward-facing Dog Stretch. The movements must be done in conjunction with the Ujjayi breath or else you will become very breathless.

If you suffer from high blood pressure, ensure that you do not bend too far forwards. If you have back problems, do not bend too far backwards and ensure that you keep your knees bent on the forward bends.

METHOD

1 Stand in the **Mountain Posture** (*Tadasana*), with your feet together and your inner thighs pulled tightly towards each other. Place your hands in the prayer position in front of your sternum. Take a preparatory breath, in and out.

2 Tighten your buttock muscles (this protects your lower back). Inhale and stretch your arms forward and up above your head, bringing your hands together, with the palms facing each other.

3 Exhale and move into the **Standing Forward Bend** (*Uttanasana*). Relax your neck so that the crown of your head points down towards the floor. If necessary, bend your knees slightly to take pressure off the back of your legs.

4 As you inhale, take your right leg back and rest the right knee on the floor (this releases pressure on the lower spine). Look up and stretch.

5 On the next exhalation, take your left leg back and place your left foot next to your right foot. At this stage only the hands and feet are on the floor, with the arms strong and straight. Keep your buttocks and knees tight and your spine straight, to protect your lower back. This is called the **Plank**. Inhale.

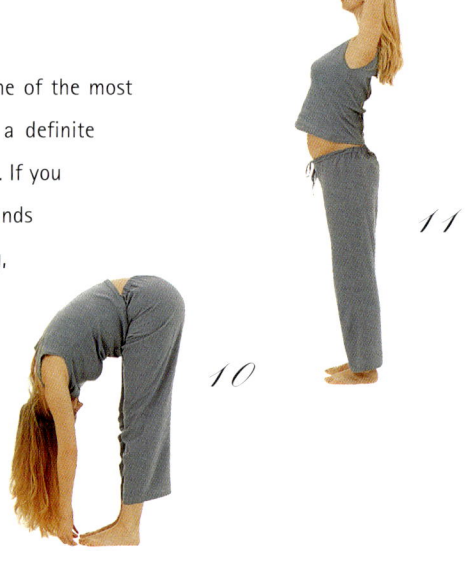

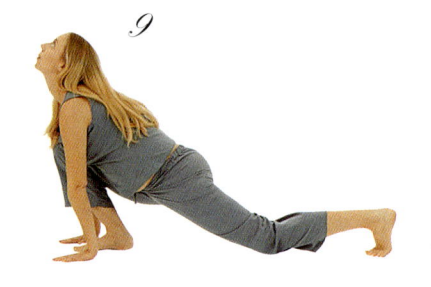

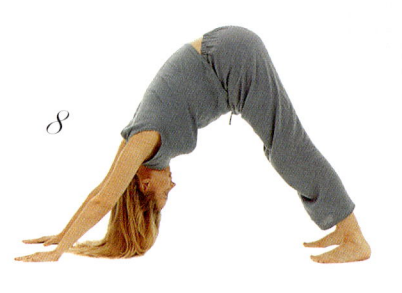

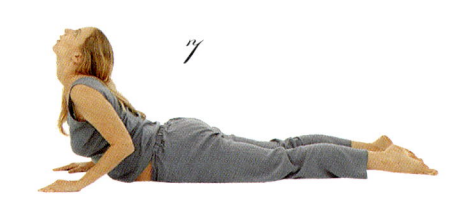

Salute to the Sun

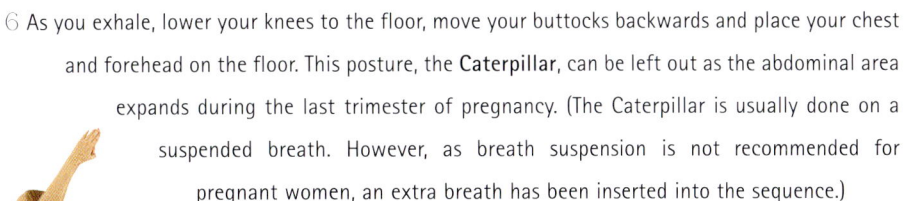

6 As you exhale, lower your knees to the floor, move your buttocks backwards and place your chest and forehead on the floor. This posture, the **Caterpillar**, can be left out as the abdominal area expands during the last trimester of pregnancy. (The Caterpillar is usually done on a suspended breath. However, as breath suspension is not recommended for pregnant women, an extra breath has been inserted into the sequence.)

7 Inhale and move into the **Cobra** *(Bhujangasana)*, sliding your hips forwards and down, until they rest on the floor. Raise your head and chest. Keep your elbows bent and tucked tightly into your ribcage. Relax your shoulders and look up. (This posture can be left out during the last trimester.)

8 Exhale, tuck your toes under and push back on your hands, raising your hips and tailbone upwards, into the **Downward-facing Dog Stretch** *(Adho Mukha Svanasana)*. Do not move your hands or feet. Straighten your arms and knees, relax your neck and try to get your heels onto the floor.

9 Inhale. Bring your right foot forwards between your hands, resting the knee on the floor. Stretch and look up.

10 Exhale and step forward with your left foot, placing it alongside the right foot, moving back into the **Standing Forward Bend** *(Uttanasana)*. Keep your knees bent if necessary to avoid putting undue pressure on the small of your back or on your legs.

11 Inhale and stretch your hands forwards and up above your head, bringing your palms together.

12 On the final exhalation, come into an upright position and bring your hands back into the prayer position.

Take a recovery breath and do the sequence again. This time take your left foot back in step 4 and bring it forward in step 9. This comprises one complete round of Salute to the Sun. As you get fitter you should be able to do 10 rounds of *Surya Namaskar* without getting breathless.

COUNTER-POSTURE Stand with your feet 30cm (18in) apart and drop into a floppy forward bend until your heart beat and breathing have returned to normal. It is essential to relax in the *Savasana*, the Pose of the Corpse (see p26) for at least five minutes and to practise deep breathing after doing the Salute to the Sun.

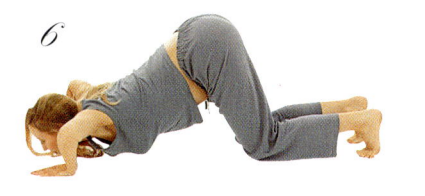

INVERTED, *or upside-down, postures revitalize the whole system. They take the weight off your legs, improve circulation, bring blood to the head and brain, and nourish body tissues. Sluggish internal organs are activated and the heart and digestive system are given a well-deserved rest.*

Relaxing in an anti-gravity position helps to reduce tension, lengthens the spine and counteracts the ageing effects of gravity.

Inverted postures work on the crown chakra, affecting the pineal gland, which is associated with higher states of awareness. The pituitary gland, which affects the functioning of all other glands, and the thyroid, which regulates metabolism, also benefit from inverted postures.

If you have never done yoga before, you should only attempt the Fountain posture from this section. Experienced yoga practitioners should practise inverted postures with caution during pregnancy, and use a chair, wall or partner for support. Avoid inverted postures entirely in your last trimester, and if you suffer from high blood pressure or a heart condition.

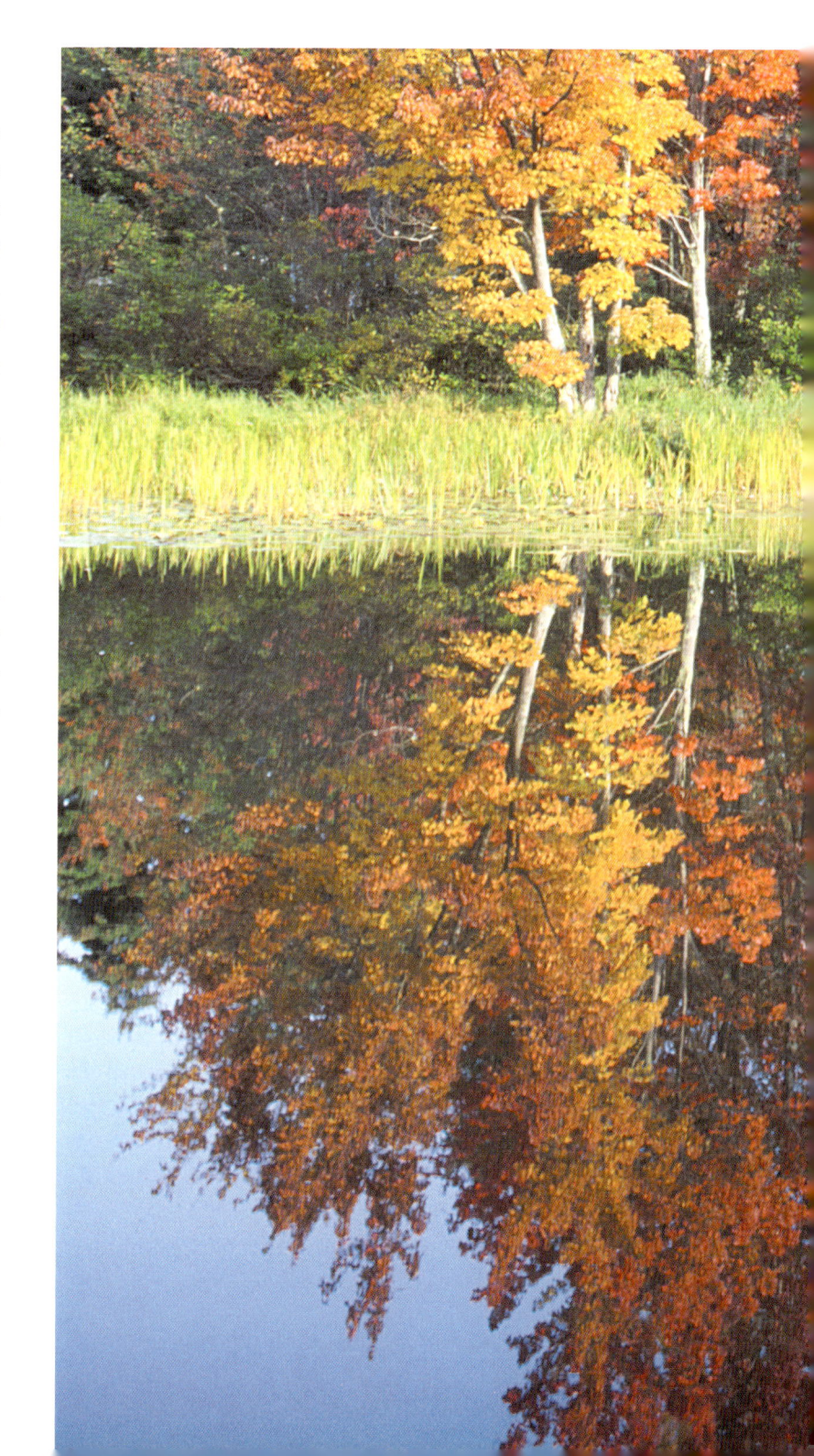

Inverted Postures

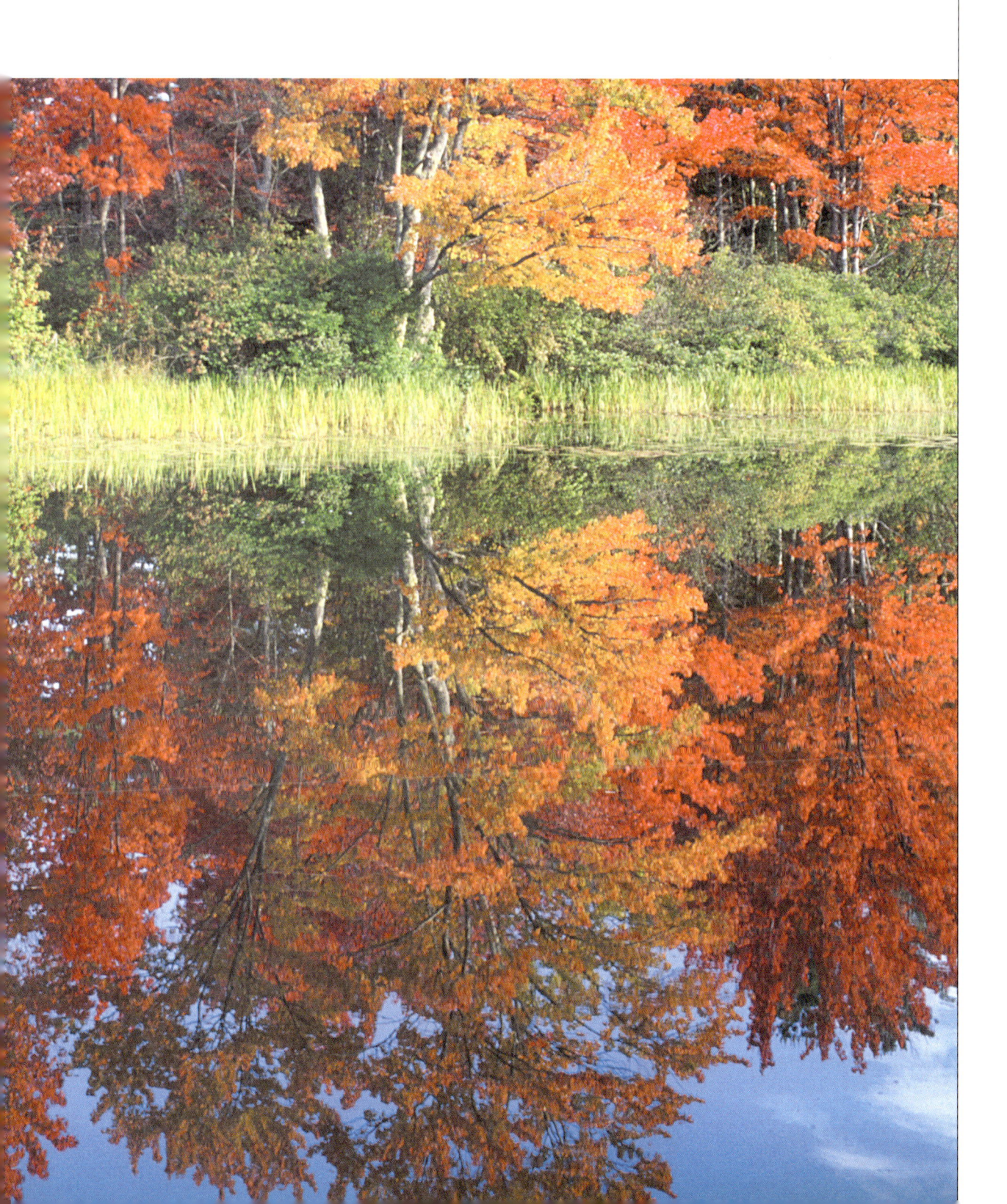

Inverted Postures

The Fountain
Viparita Karani

(B | 1 2 3)

BENEFITS This exceptionally relaxing posture is highly recommended for pregnant women, as it releases all the internal organs, as well as the foetus, from the pull of gravity. It assists circulation and is also good for relieving swollen veins and is excellent when you want to feel rejuvenated.

CAUTIONS Normally you should not practise inverted postures in the last trimester, but as only the legs are raised, this caution does not apply for this posture.

METHOD Work against a wall and have two pillows close at hand. Sit on the floor with your legs stretched out and your hip against the wall (1). Lean back and sideways, placing your weight on your elbows. Swing your legs towards the wall (2), turning so that you end up lying on your back at right angles to the wall with both feet stretched up towards the ceiling. Wiggle your buttocks as close to the wall as possible.

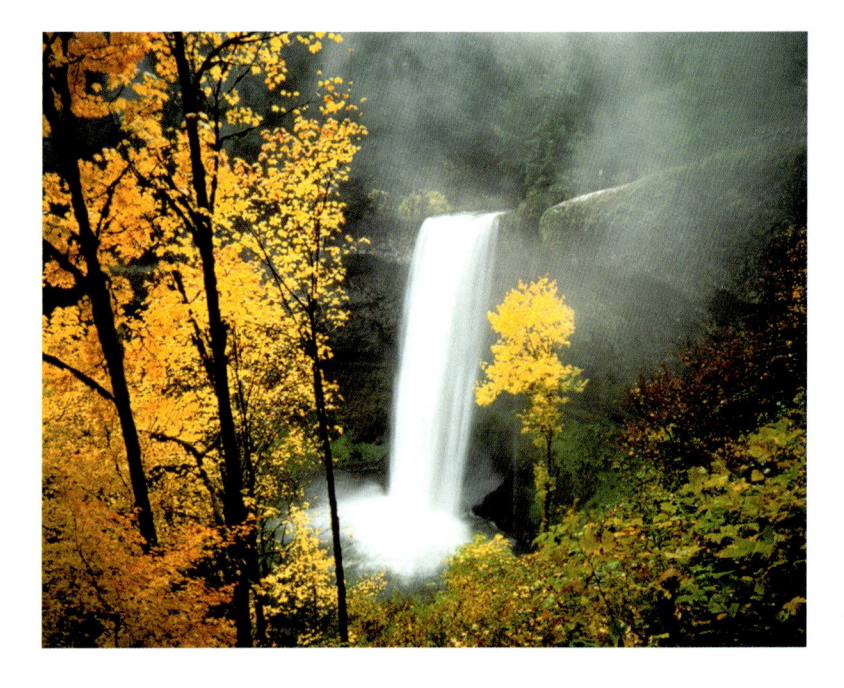

Bend your knees and place both feet on the wall. Push against the wall with your feet, raise your hips to place the two pillows underneath them, so that the pillows and your buttocks all touch the wall. Now, lower your hips and buttocks down onto the pillows and straighten your legs up the wall towards the ceiling again (3). Stretch your arms along the floor next to your body, close your eyes and just relax.

To come out of the posture, bend your knees and roll over onto your right-hand side. Rest for a moment, and then place your left hand on the floor in front of you, pushing yourself up into a sitting position.

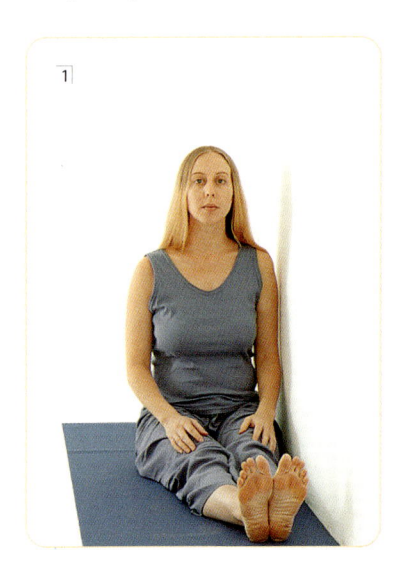

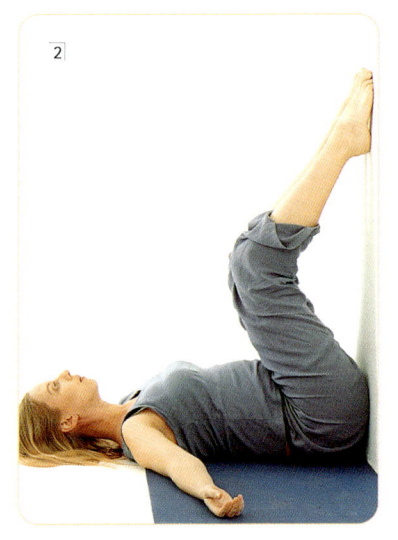

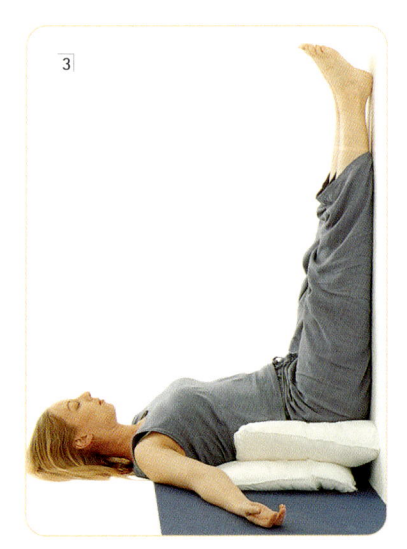

Downward-facing Dog Stretch

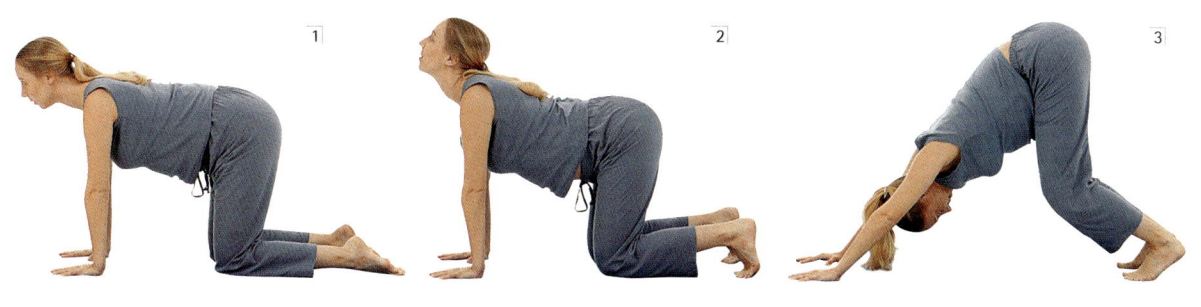

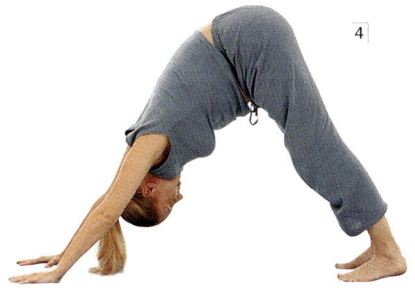

Downward-facing Dog Stretch

Adho Mukha Svanasana

(1 | 2)

BENEFITS This posture releases the neck and shoulder muscles and stretches the hamstrings. It strengthens the entire body.

CAUTIONS Avoid this posture if you suffer from high blood pressure. Do not practise inverted postures in the last trimester.

METHOD Kneel on all fours with your hands directly underneath your shoulders and the fingers spread wide apart (1). Ensure that your middle fingers are parallel to each other. Have your knees directly underneath your hips with your feet parallel to each other. Tuck your toes under, drop your belly button down towards the floor and inhale (2). As you exhale, push back on your hands, raising your tailbone towards the ceiling (3). Straighten your legs and lower your heels to the floor (4). Ensure that your breathing is regular and even, and hold the pose for as long as it is comfortable. (This is easier said than done if you are new to yoga.) However, it will eventually become a wonderfully relaxing posture, so give yourself time to get used to it.

If your hamstrings are tight, then inhale and straighten the right knee as far as it will go (keeping that heel on the floor, if possible) and bend the left knee. As you exhale, bend the right knee and straighten the left. Keep alternating the legs as you bend and stretch them.

To come out of the posture, bend your knees, place your buttocks on your heels and rest your forehead on the floor or on your fists.

COUNTER-POSTURE Pose of the Child (see p40).

VARIATION

Come into the Cat Stretch position (see p46). Inhale and raise your head and tailbone as you drop your navel. Arch your back and exhale. Inhale, raising your head and tailbone and dropping your navel as you tuck your toes under. When you exhale, lift your knees off the floor and move into the Downward-facing Dog Stretch. Hold this posture for a full inhalation and exhalation. On the next inhalation, move into the Cat Stretch and restart the sequence. Your body should move rhythmically with your breath. The entire sequence moves to a count of three. In the Cat Stretch, the first inhalation is the first count, the exhalation is the second count and the inhalation is the third count. Exhaling into the Dog Stretch is the first count, the inhalation (while holding the Dog Stretch) is the second count and the exhalation (still holding the Dog Stretch) is the third count. This makes it easier to get the rhythm of the movement.

Inverted Postures

The Shoulder Stand

Sarvangasana

1 | 2

BENEFITS The Shoulder Stand is said to be the mother of all yoga postures because it brings about a feeling of general wellbeing. It balances the thyroid gland and keeps the spine supple. It also releases the internal organs and the foetus from the pull of gravity.

CAUTIONS Do not practise inverted postures in the last trimester (after 30 weeks). Do not attempt this posture at all if you begin yoga only after your fifth month of pregnancy. If you have been practising yoga for some time before falling pregnant, you may be confident enough to do the shoulder stand until your seventh month if you have no complications with your pregnancy. Do not turn your head to the side.

METHOD Lie on your back (1) and draw your knees up onto your chest (2). Have your arms on the floor alongside your body with the palms facing downwards. Inhale and as you exhale lift your hips off the floor and push down on your hands, bringing the knees onto the forehead. Quickly bend your elbows and place your hands underneath your hips (3) to take the weight as you straighten your legs up towards the ceiling. This is called the Half Shoulder Stand. Bring your elbows as close to each other as possible. This will ensure a comfortable position. Keep your legs together. Now, push your hips forwards with your fingertips, taking your hands closer towards your bra strap. This will raise the body up into a straight line (4). Tighten your buttock muscles for the first couple of breaths of the posture and then allow your body to relax into the pose. Keep up a regular and even breathing rhythm and close your eyes.

Hold the posture for as long as it is comfortable. If you are able to stay there for longer than two minutes you should experience a wonderful feeling of floating, or of being suspended from the ceiling. To come out of the posture, bend your knees onto your forehead and slowly roll down onto the floor. Just lie there for a while to enjoy the benefits of the

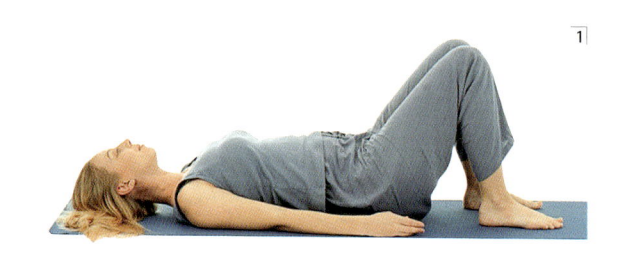

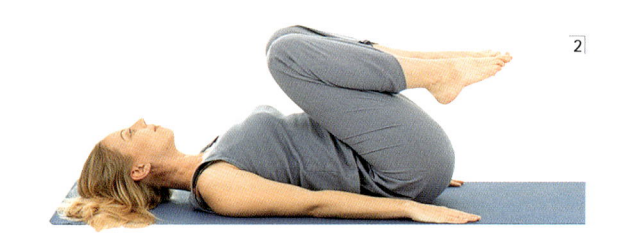

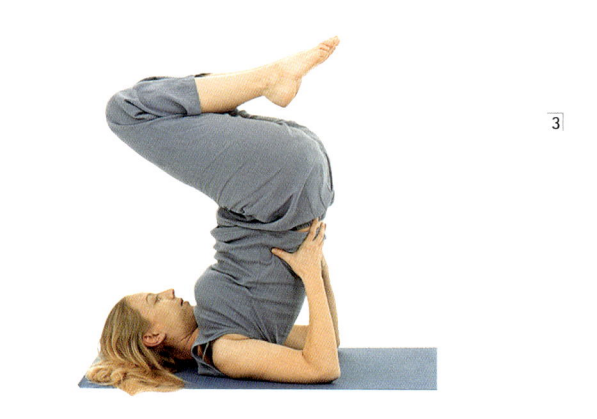

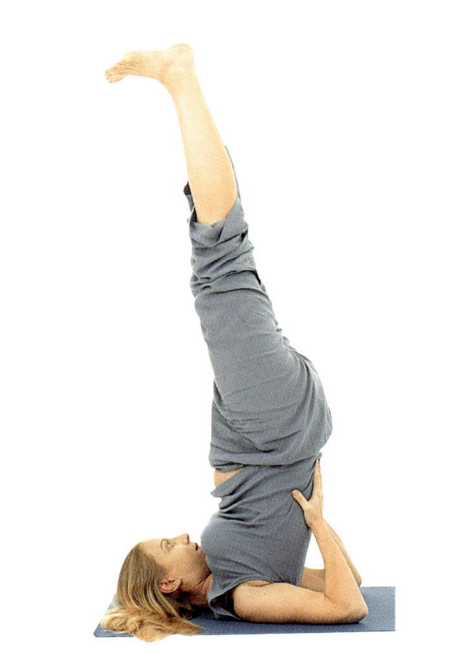

The Shoulder Stand

posture before doing the counter-position. Sometimes the vertebrae at the base of the neck push into the floor. If this occurs, place a folded blanket or towel underneath your shoulders and back. The blanket should come to the top of the shoulders and the head should rest on the floor.

COUNTER-POSTURE The Fish (see p57).

VARIATION

Sit on the floor with your legs stretched out and your left hip close to the wall (1). Lean back on your right elbow and swing your legs up the wall (2), turning so that your back is at right angles to the wall. Bend your knees and place the soles of your feet on the wall (3). Press against the wall with your feet and raise your hips (4). Place your hands under your hips (5) and stretch your legs, resting your heels against the wall (6). Breathe gently and evenly. To come out of the posture, bend your knees and take your weight back onto your feet. Lower your buttocks to the floor. Bring your knees onto your chest and roll over onto your right side. Rest for a moment or two before placing your left hand on the floor in-front of you and pushing yourself up into a sitting position.

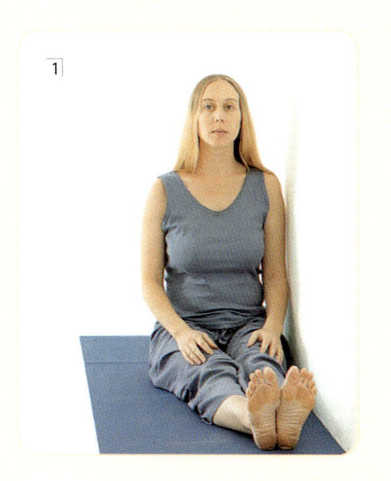

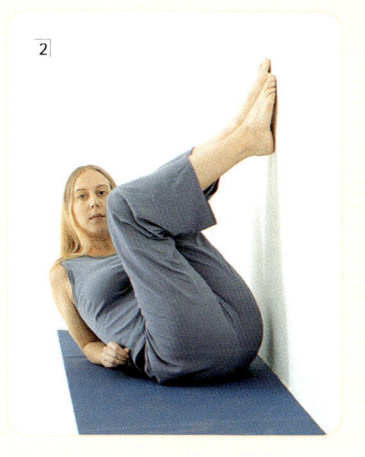

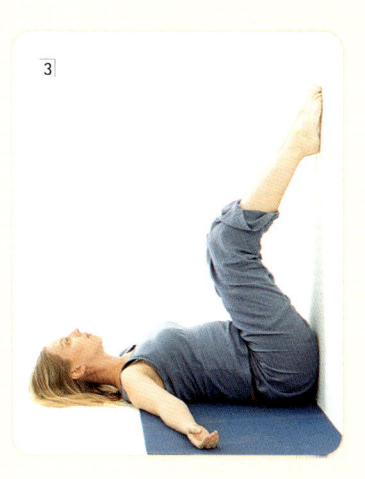

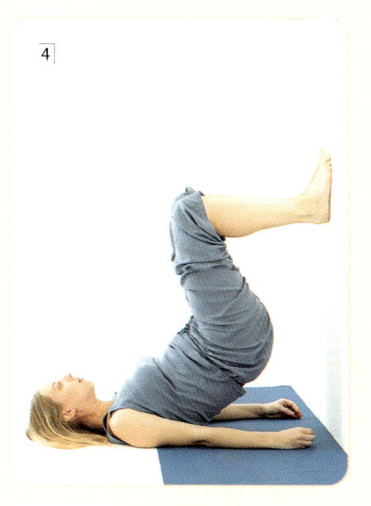

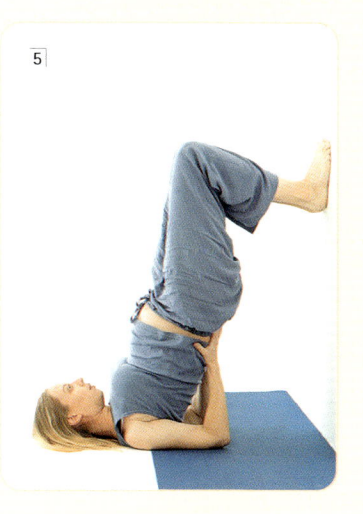

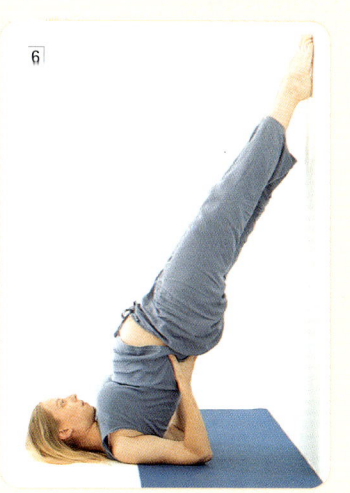

Inverted Postures

The Plough

Halasana

| 1 | 2 |

BENEFITS Activates the pituitary gland (see p14), massages the abdominal organs, keeps the spine supple and stretches the back muscles, shoulders and hamstrings.

CAUTIONS Do not attempt this posture unless you are able to do the Shoulder Stand comfortably. Do not turn your head. As your pregnancy advances it may become necessary to keep your legs slightly apart and rest your feet on a chair (see right). Do not practise inverted postures in the last trimester (after 30 weeks).

METHOD Begin by going into the Shoulder Stand (1–3). Once in the Shoulder Stand, with your spine supported by your hands, inhale and, as you exhale, slowly take your legs and feet over your head until they touch the ground (4). If your feet do not reach the ground, then rest them on a chair.

Stretch your hands away from you behind your back and interlace your fingers. Roll your shoulder blades closer together. Try to keep your palms touching each other and your elbows straight. This will stretch the shoulders. Place your little fingers on the floor if possible.

Try to keep your spine straight. Straighten your knees and push your heels down towards the floor. Relax into the posture. Close your eyes and hold the position for as long as it remains comfortable. To come out of the posture, bend your knees and support your hips with your hands as you slowly roll down onto the floor. Alternately, go back up into the Shoulder Stand and notice how doing the Plough improves your Shoulder Stand.

COUNTER-POSTURE The Fish (p57) or the Cat Stretch (p46).

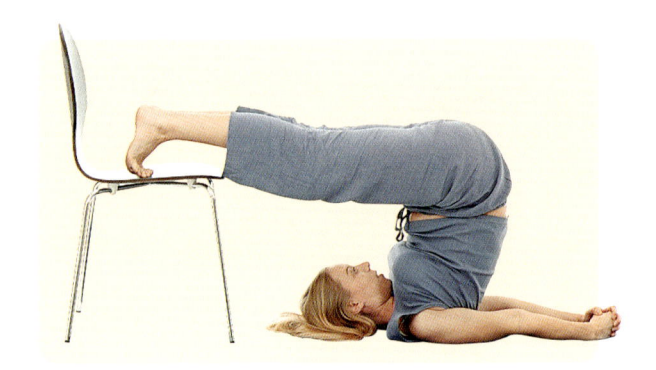

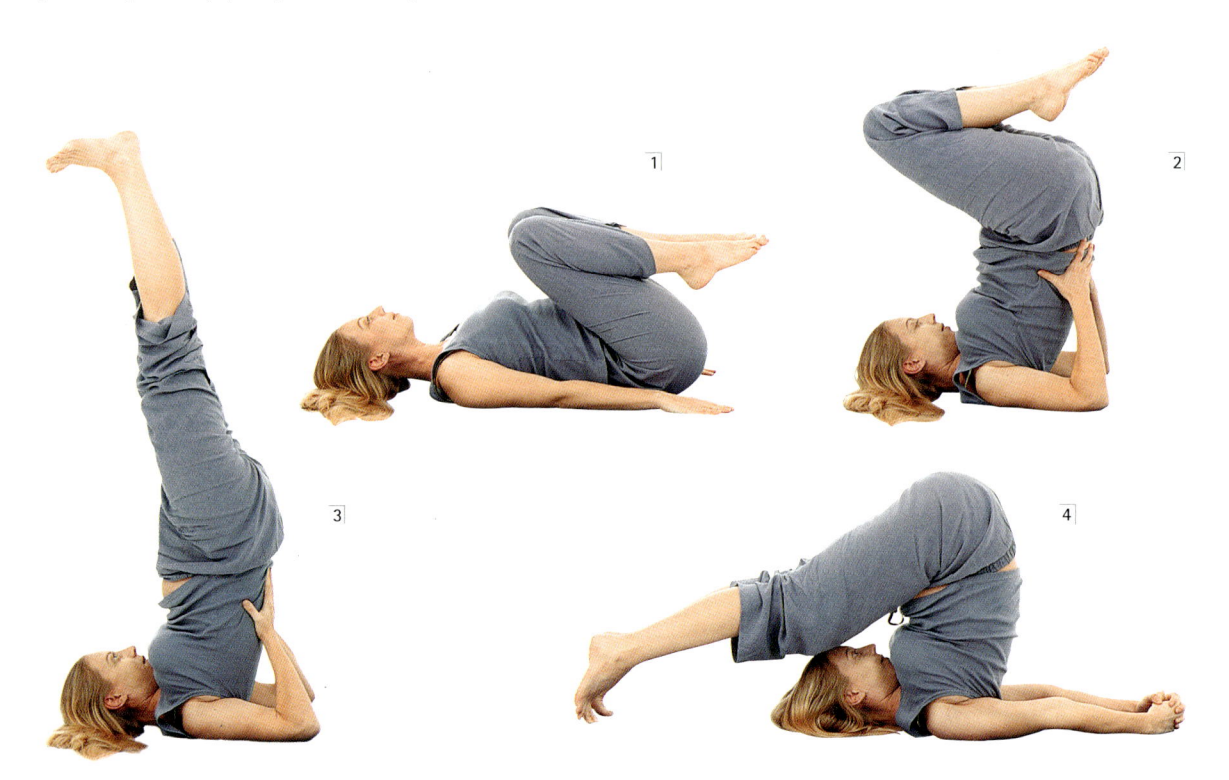

The Little Headstand

Salamba Sirsasana

B 1 2

BENEFITS Brings oxygenated blood to the brain, face and throat. Releases the internal organs and the foetus from the pull of gravity.

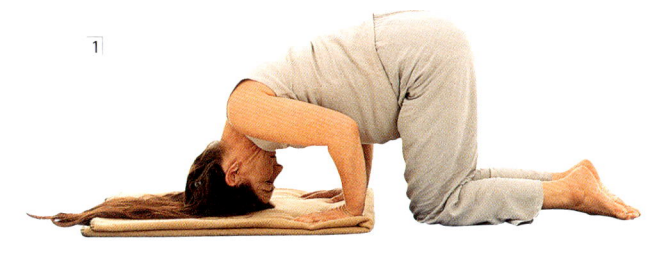

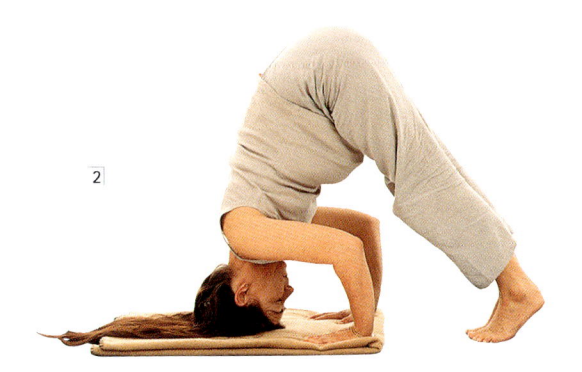

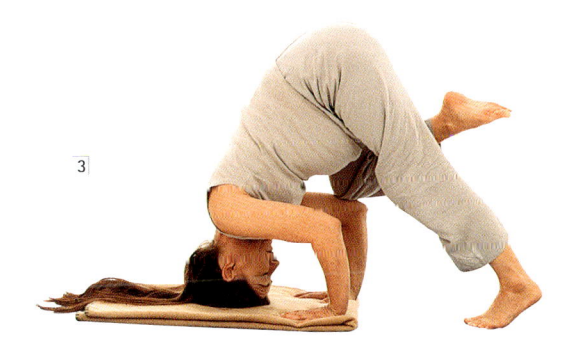

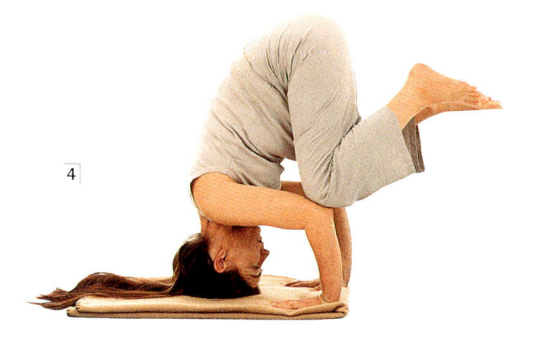

CAUTIONS Do not do headstands if you have a neck problem. When you practise this posture, it is essential that you are on the crown of your head. To find this, hold the tips of your ears between your fingers and thumbs. Run your index fingers straight up your head and they will meet at the crown. The Little Headstand is much easier than it looks, but before practising it at home, ask your yoga teacher to assist you in class until you are comfortable with it. At home, have a partner on hand to support you until you feel confident.

Do not practise inverted postures in the last trimester (after 30 weeks) and do not attempt this posture at all if you only start yoga after your fifth month of pregnancy.

METHOD Place a folded blanket on your mat (or against a wall for added safety). The area covered by the blanket must be large enough to accommodate your head and hands, as it is essential that they are on the same level. Kneel in front of the blanket and place the base of your palms on the edge closest to your body. Spread your fingers wide apart and have the middle fingers parallel to each other. Place the crown of your head on the blanket so that the head and the hands form a triangle (1). This is the most important part of the posture as it provides a secure base. Straighten your legs, bringing your buttocks up into the air (2). Slowly walk your feet towards your hands. When your back is perpendicular to the floor, bend your right knee and rest it on the top of your right elbow, lifting the foot off the floor (3). Bend the left knee and rest it on top of your left elbow, lifting the foot up. Relax the weight of your legs onto your elbows (4). It is necessary for the elbows to be absolutely perpendicular to the floor to bear this weight. Make sure you are not holding your breath. To come out of the posture, place your feet back on the floor, return to a kneeling position with your buttocks on your heels and forehead on the floor.

Do not be afraid of this posture. Although it looks difficult, it is very simple to do.

COUNTER-POSTURE After doing the Little Headstand, it is essential to rest in the Pose of the Child (p40) before lifting your head, otherwise you might get dizzy or light headed.

Inverted Postures

THE HEADSTAND
Sirsasana

A 1 2

BENEFITS The Headstand is said to be the father of all the yoga postures. It brings oxygenated blood to the brain, eyes, nose, throat and face and releases the internal organs and the foetus from gravity.

CAUTIONS You must balance on the crown of your head. Do not attempt the Headstand if you have neck problems. Ask your teacher to assist you in class until you are comfortable with it and use a partner to support you at home. Do not do inverted postures in the last trimester. Do not do headstands at all if you only begin yoga after your fifth month or later.

METHOD Kneel and place your hands on a folded blanket, as for the Little Headstand. Straighten your legs and walk your feet towards your hands until your spine is erect (1–2). Bend and raise your right leg, drawing the knee towards your chest (3), then bend and raise your left knee (4). Hold this posture and take a breath. As you exhale, extend your legs slowly, straightening them towards the ceiling (5). Tighten your buttock muscles, keeping your breathing even and gentle. Hold the posture for as long as it is comfortable. To come down, bend the knees and bring them back towards your chest, then place your feet on the floor. Rest with your buttocks on your heels and your forehead on the floor.

If you feel nervous about the Headstand, try it against the wall or, even better, get a partner to assist you by placing his or her knee against the small of your back to stop you from rolling over. Your partner can also hold your feet.

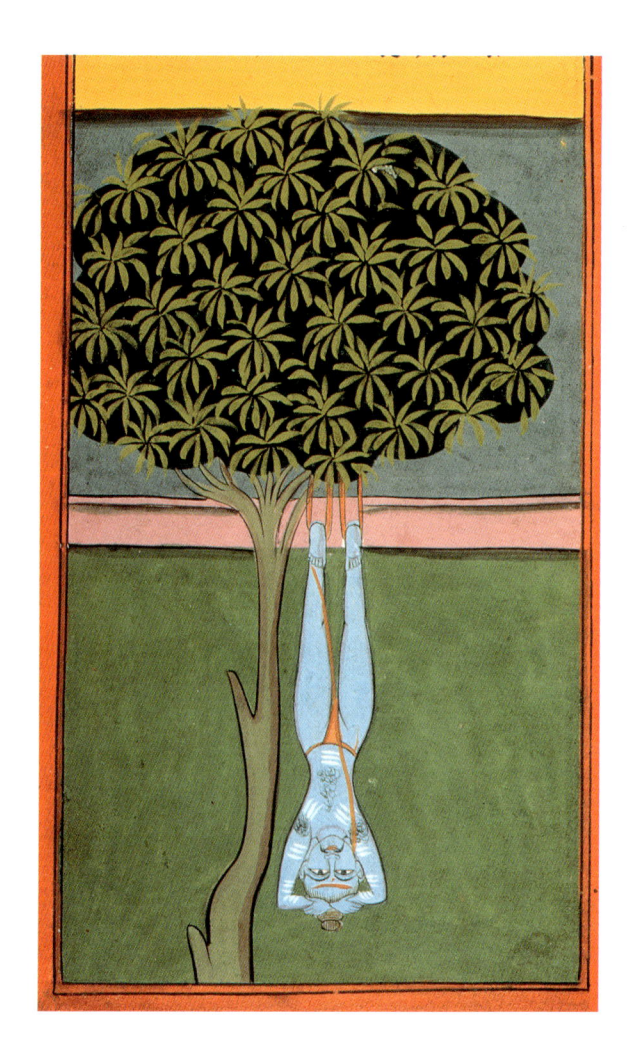

COUNTER-POSTURE Rest in the Pose of the Child (p40) before your raise your head to avoid becoming dizzy.

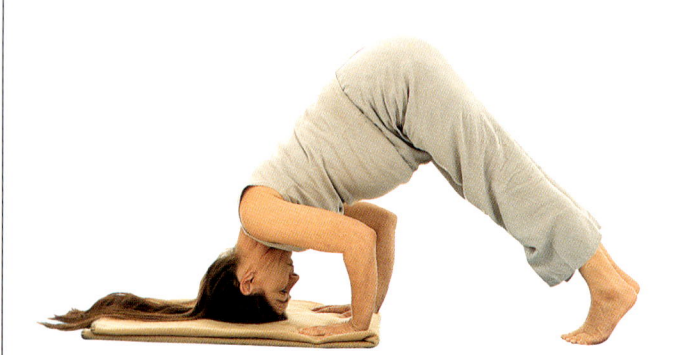

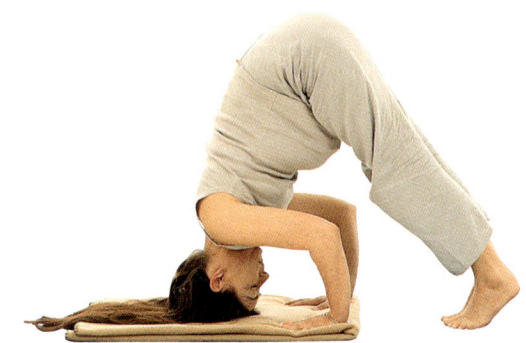

1

2

The Headstand

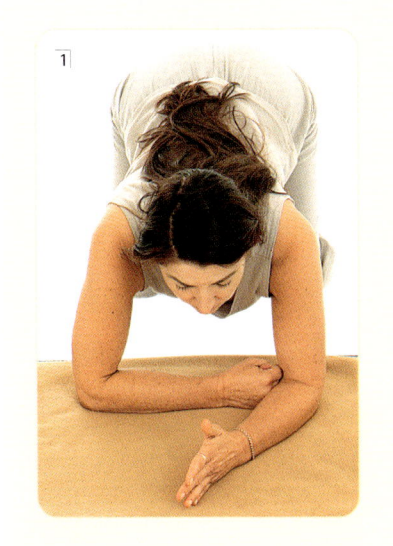

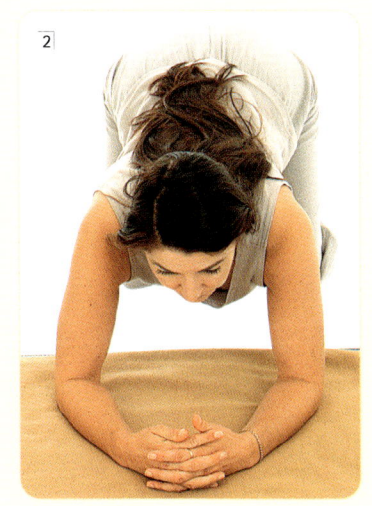

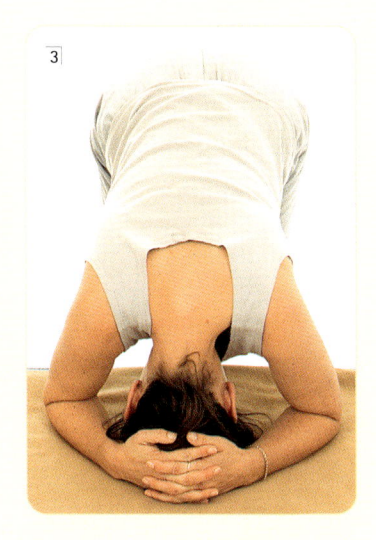

VARIATION

This is an alternative way to place your head and hands and may make you feel more stable. Kneeling, place your left elbow on a blanket. Make a fist with your right hand and place it against your left elbow (1). Keeping the right elbow in line with the left elbow, join your hands and interlace your fingers (2). Do not move your elbows as you do this. Place the back of your head into the curve formed by your hands, ensuring that the crown is on the floor (3). Proceed with the Headstand as described opposite.

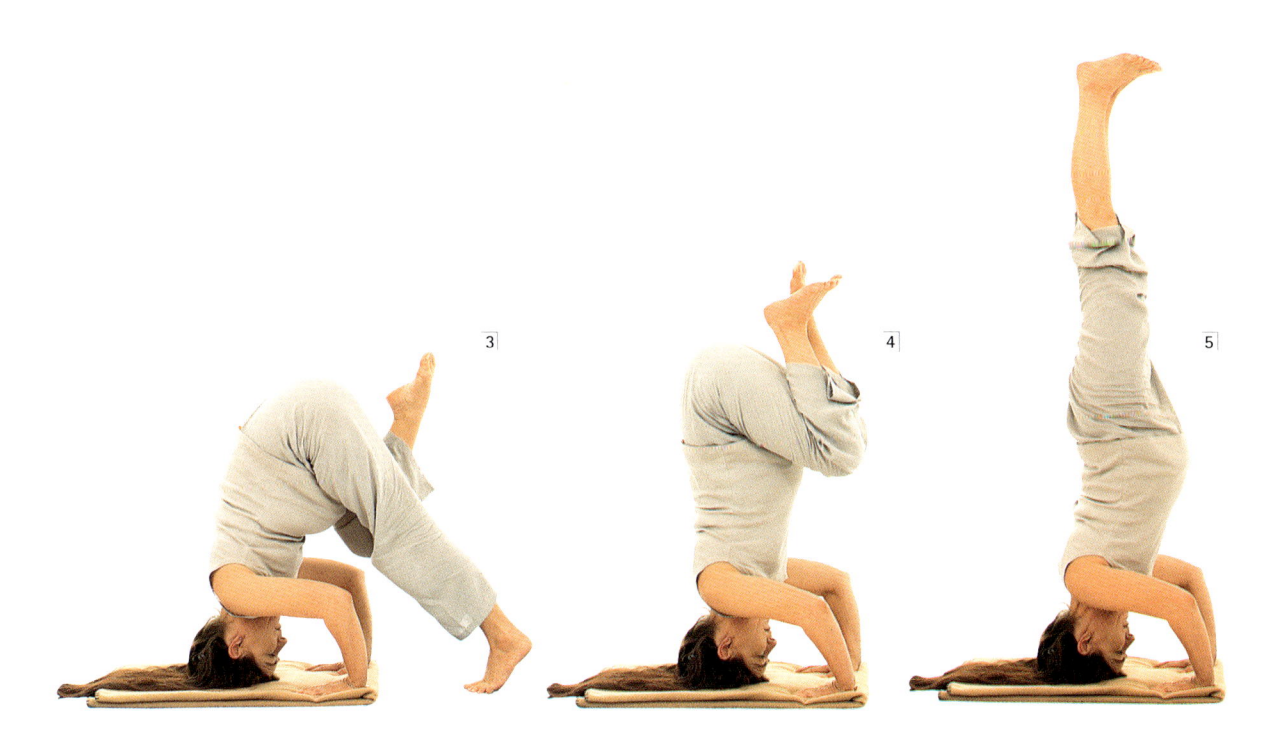

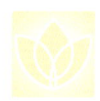

IT IS *advisable to rest for at least four to six weeks between giving birth and recommencing an exercise routine. You will probably be so busy with your new baby that it will be difficult to find the time to exercise, but it is important to get your body back into shape. As your muscles contract back into their original state they need to be strengthened. Your doctor or midwife will indicate when it is safe for you to begin exercising again.*

All the postures given in this book can be practised after birth. However, those in this chapter will help to strengthen the abdominal muscles in particular. Work at your own pace and allow your body to dictate your progress.

An advantage of continuing yoga after giving birth is that your hips and groin are very flexible and open, making it easier to achieve postures. Regular yoga practice also helps you to cope with the demands of motherhood, such as sleeplessness, mood shifts as your hormone balance alters, and the challenge of caring for a new baby.

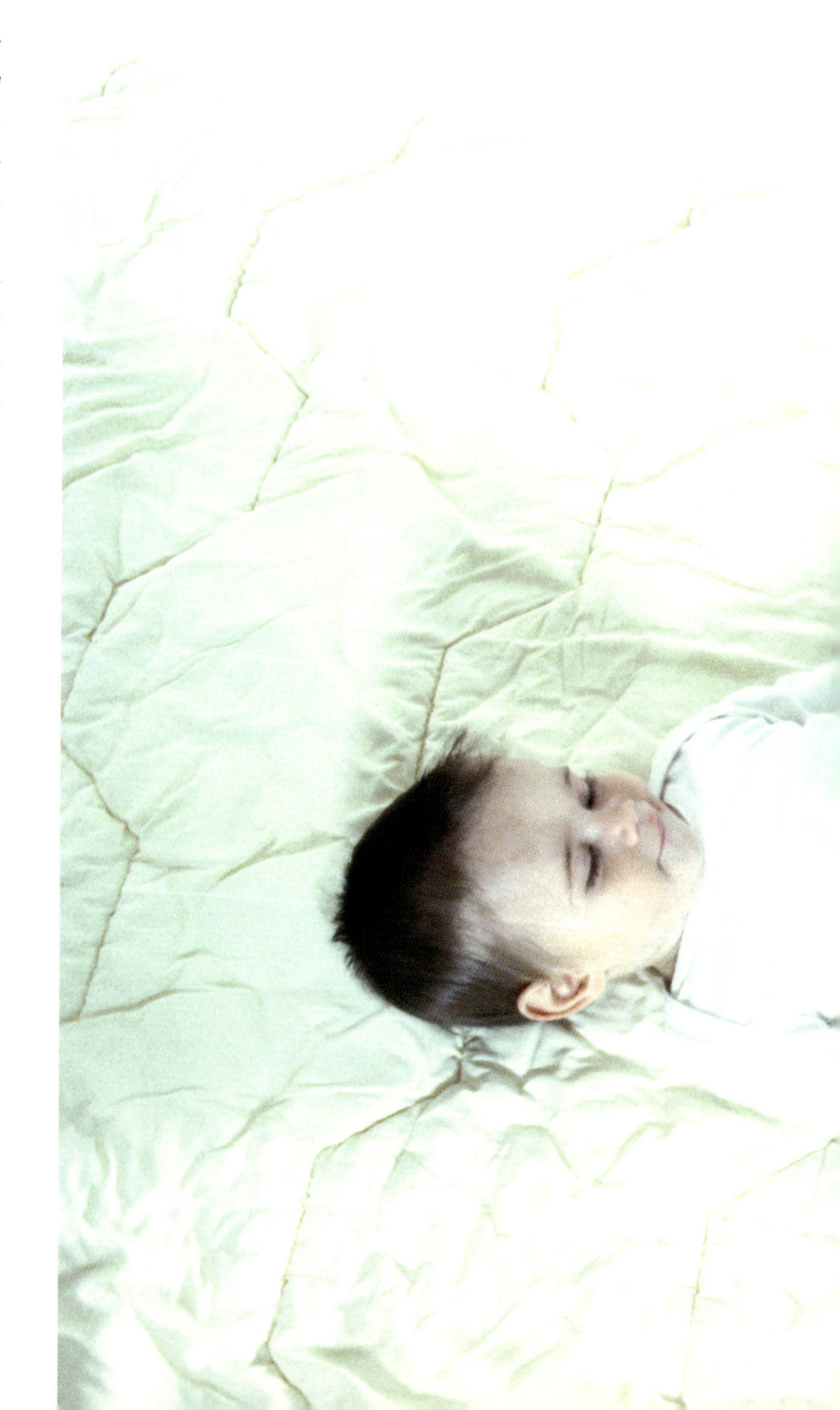

Postnatal Postures

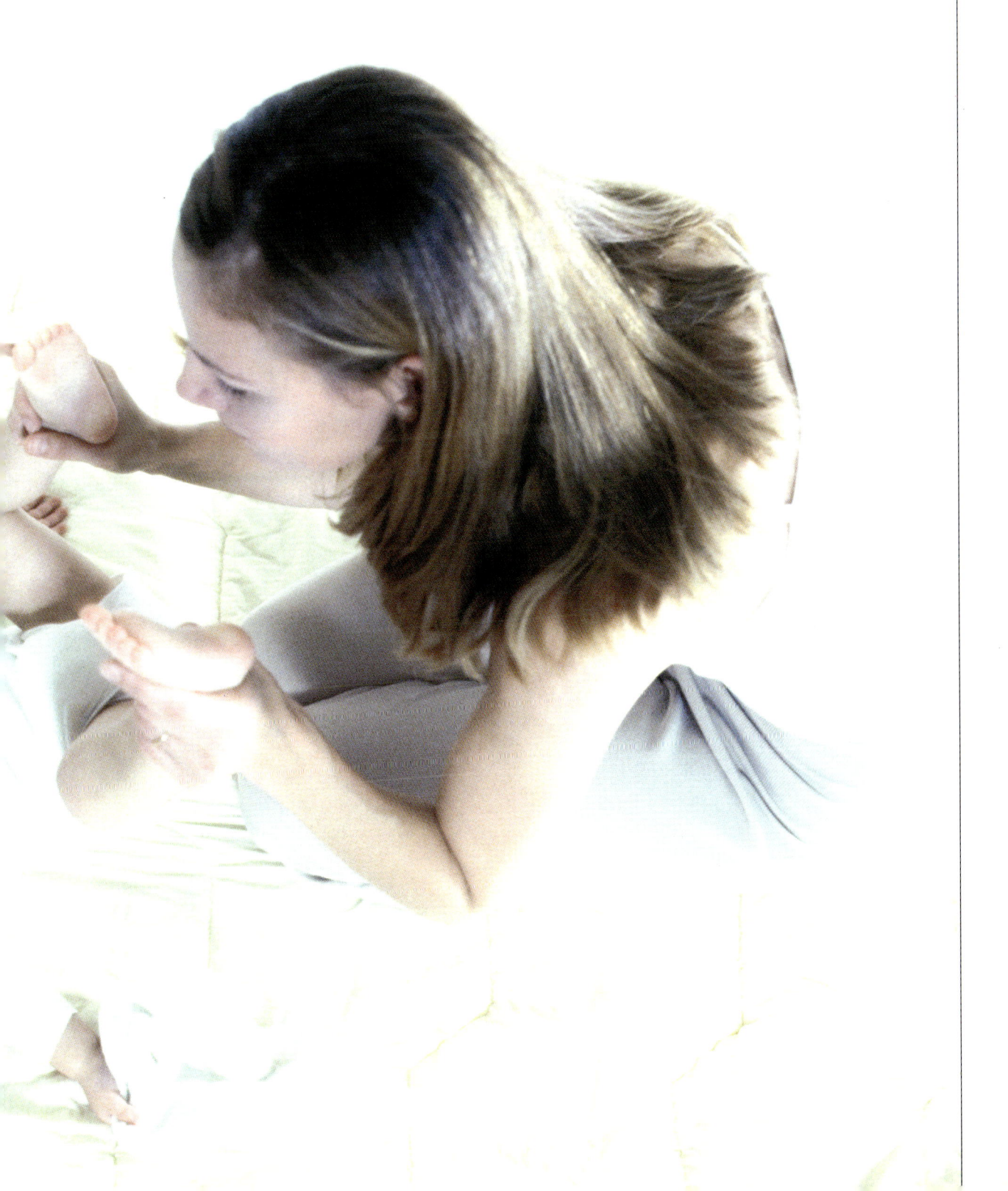

Postnatal Postures

Curl Ups
(Beginner)

BENEFITS Strengthens the abdominal (stomach) muscles.

METHOD Lie flat on your back and draw your knees onto your chest. Interlace your fingers behind your head (1). Inhale, and as you exhale, slowly lift your head and touch your right elbow to your right knee. Inhale and slowly lower your head and elbows onto the floor. Repeat this three more times. Take the left elbow to the left knee four times. Then touch the right elbow to the left knee four times (2), and the left elbow to the right knee four times. Lastly, touch both elbows to both knees four times (3). Ensure that you always lift the head on an exhalation and lower the head and elbows on an inhalation. The more slowly you can do this posture the more beneficial it will be to your stomach muscles. Use Ujjayi breathing when you do this exercise.

COUNTER-POSTURE Lie flat and stretch your legs out along the floor, with your hands at your sides. Inhale and push your stomach muscles up towards the ceiling. As you exhale, expel the air out of your mouth and drop your stomach muscles back into a relaxed position (think of pricking a balloon with a pin – everything just deflates). Repeat the movement twice more.

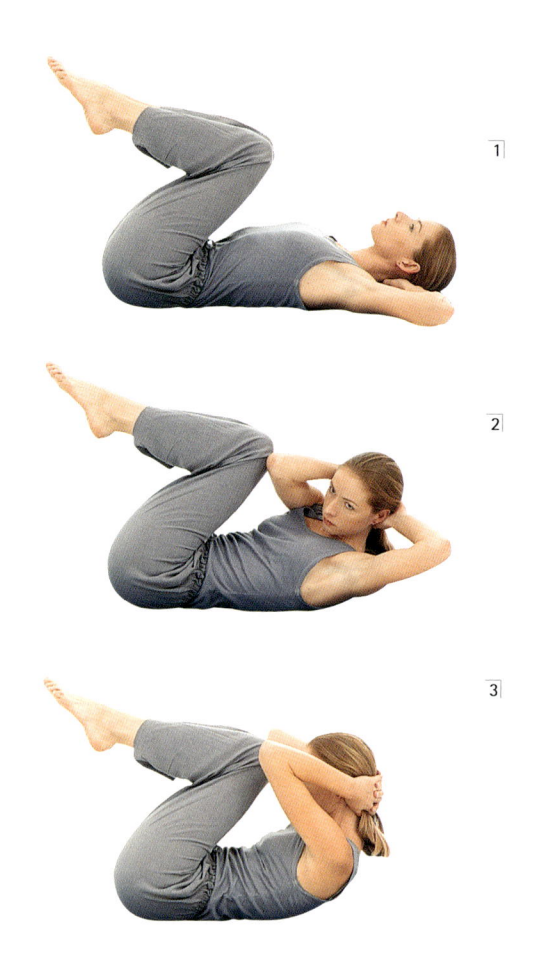

Stomach Clenching
(Intermediate)

BENEFITS This strenuous exercise strengthens the stomach muscles. It is also excellent for releasing tension from the small of the back.

METHOD Lie flat on your back with your legs outstretched. Inhale, flex your feet (1) and make fists with your hands. As you exhale, raise your head, shoulders and arms off the floor (2), keeping your legs and lower back in contact with the floor. Do not stop breathing. Hold the posture for six breaths and then lower yourself back to the floor. Repeat two or three times.

COUNTER-POSTURE Inhale and expand your stomach muscles towards the ceiling, releasing them on the exhalation.

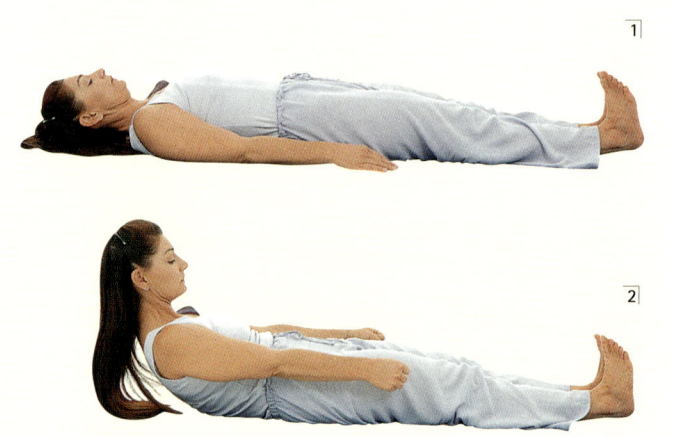

Buttock Balance

Navasana

(Intermediate)

BENEFITS Strengthens the abdominal (stomach) muscles.

CAUTIONS Do not round your spine. Keep the sternum (breastbone) lifted or you will lose your balance.

METHOD Sit on your mat with your knees bent and your feet on the floor in front of you. Place your hands underneath your knees and hold your left wrist with your right hand (1). Lift your sternum. Inhale and lift your feet 20cm (8in) off the floor (2). As you exhale, straighten your legs so that they are at a 45-degree angle to the floor and your body is in the shape of a 'V' (3).

It is difficult to breathe in this posture if you are not used to it, so focus on your breathing. As you exhale, release your hands from under your knees, stretching them out in front of you (4), and hold the posture for as long as it is comfortable. To come out of the posture, support your legs behind the knees, bend them and place your feet back on the floor. Repeat three or four times.

COUNTER-POSTURE Lie flat on your back and expand your stomach muscles up towards the ceiling as you breathe in. Breathe out through your mouth as you relax again. Repeat a few times.

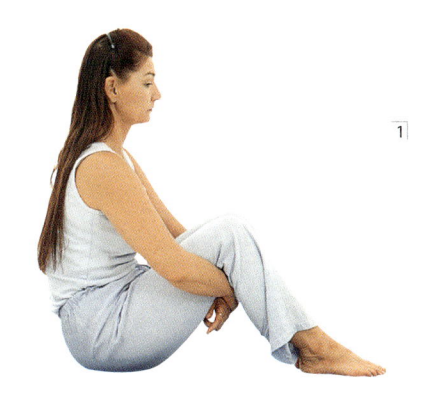

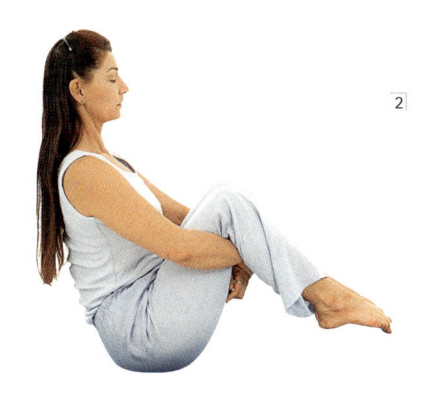

VARIATION

(Intermediate)

METHOD Go into Navasana (4) and take hold of your insteps or toes with your hands. If you cannot reach your feet then hold onto your ankles. Keeping hold of your feet, straighten your legs and open your legs wide. Keep your sternum lifted and spine straight. Hold the posture for as long as is comfortable. To come out of the posture, bring your legs together, release your feet and lower them to the floor.

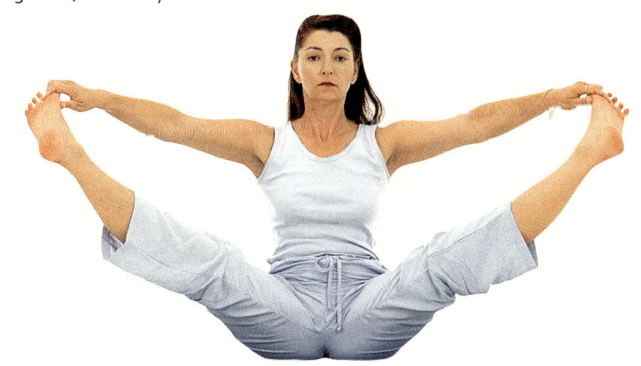

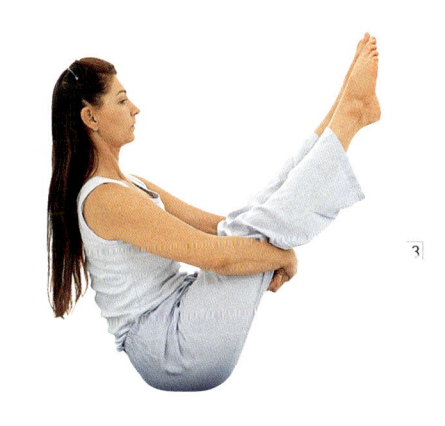

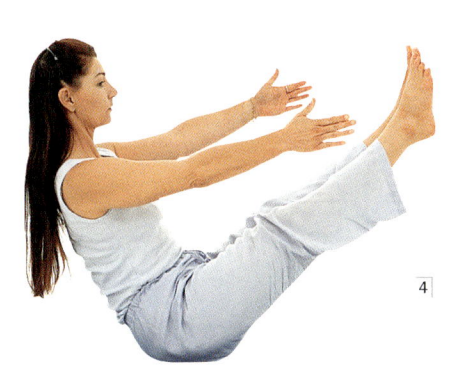

Postnatal Postures

THE CANDLE
(Intermediate)

BENEFITS Strengthens the abdominal (stomach) muscles and the hips.

CAUTIONS If you suffer from back problems, do not lower your legs slowly to the floor to come out of the posture. Rather, bend your knees onto your chest and then place your feet back on the floor.

METHOD Lie flat on your back with your knees over your chest. Keeping your head on the floor, interlace your fingers behind your head (1). Inhale, and as you exhale, extend your feet up towards the ceiling (2). Push the small of your back firmly into the floor and draw your navel down towards your spine. The more you push your back into the floor, the easier the posture will be. Straighten your legs and flex your feet as though you are standing on the ceiling. Do not stop breathing. Hold the posture for as long as is comfortable.

To come out of the posture, exhale and lower your straight legs slowly to the floor. If this is too difficult, bend your knees to your chest and then place your feet back on the floor. In time, your stomach muscles will strengthen and you will be able to lower your legs gradually.

COUNTER-POSTURE Apanasana (p39) will release the tension exerted on the abdominal muscles and lower back, allowing them to relax.

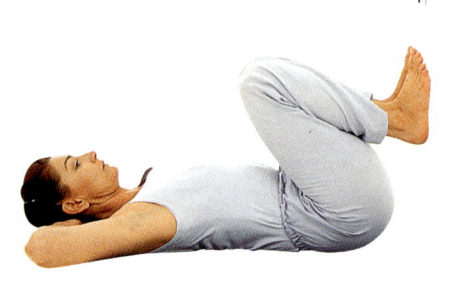

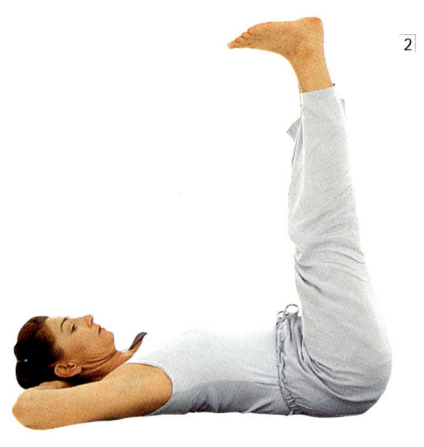

VARIATION 1
(Intermediate)

Go into the Candle. On an inhalation, slowly open your legs as wide as you can. As you exhale, bring them back together again. Try to keep your legs straight and keep pushing into the heels. Remember, the harder you push the small of the back into the floor, the easier the posture becomes. Do this as many times as you can. Concentrate on breathing.

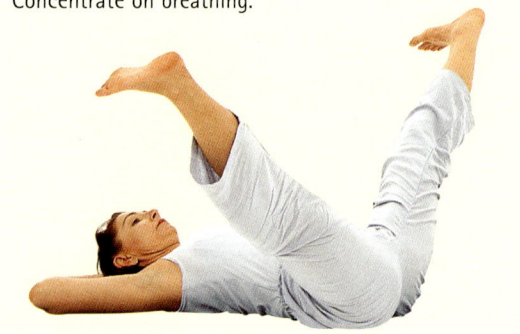

VARIATION 2
(Intermediate)

Go into the Candle, inhale and open your legs. Release your hands from behind your head, lift your head and shoulders off the floor and extend your arms through your open legs. Concentrate on your breathing and hold the position for as long as it is comfortable. To come out of it, return your head and shoulders to the floor and lower your legs.

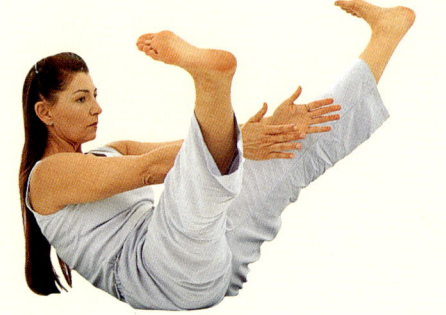

Supine Spinal Twist

Parivartanasana

(Beginners)

BENEFITS Releases tension in the lower back, brings flexibility to the spine and works the waistline.

METHOD Lie on your back with your knees over your chest and your arms outstretched at a 90-degree angle, with your palms facing downwards (1). Inhale, and as you exhale, slowly drop your knees to the floor on the right, turning your head to look at your left hand (2). Both shoulders should be flat on the floor so the twist is in your spine not your chest. Inhale and bring your head and knees slowly back to the centre. Exhale, taking your knees over to the left and turning your head to the right (3). Inhale and bring your head and knees back to the centre. Repeat seven more times to each side. Keep your knees, ankles and feet together and bring your knees as close to your armpits as possible. Do the posture dynamically, as described, or statically, keeping your knees on the floor on each side for eight breaths.

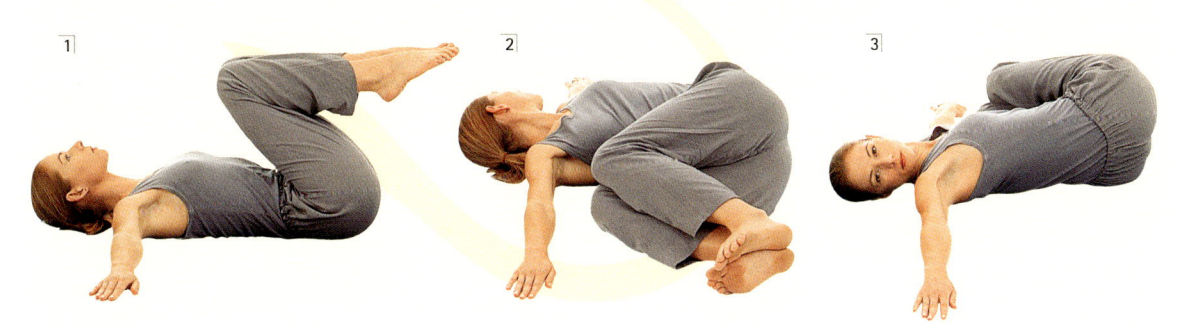

Sideways Swing

(Intermediate)

BENEFITS Wonderful for reducing the waistline as well as strengthening the abdominal muscles and hamstrings.

METHOD Kneel on your mat with your buttocks on your heels. Inhale and raise yourself into an upright kneeling position. Fold your arms across your chest (1) and hold them there for the duration of the exercise. As you exhale, lower your buttocks to the floor onto your right side (2). Inhale and come back into a raised kneeling position (3). Exhale and lower your buttocks to the floor on your left side (4). Inhale and move back into an upright kneeling position. Repeat this exercise 15 times to each side.

COUNTER-POSTURE Pose of the Child (see p40).

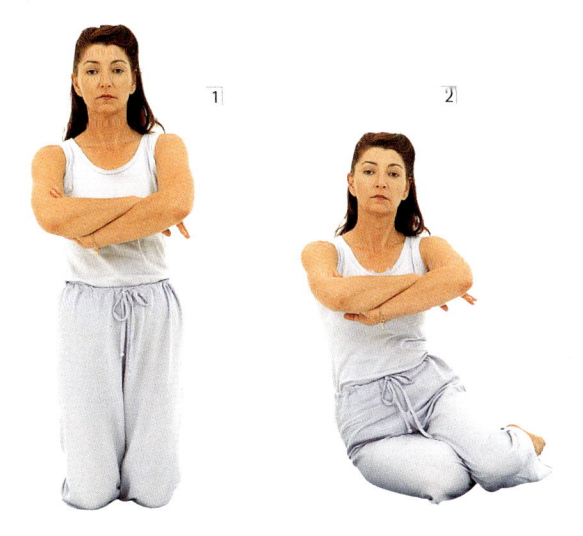

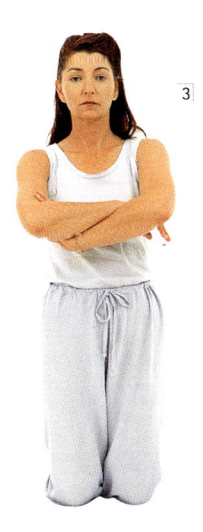

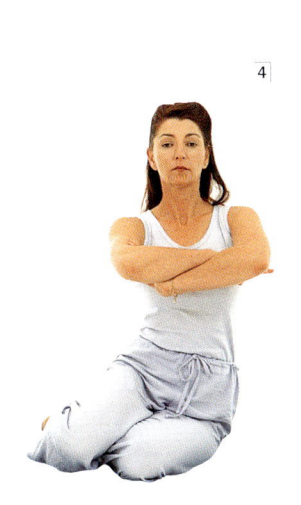

Postnatal Postures

Upright Spinal Twist

Pashasana

(Intermediate)

BENEFITS This posture brings flexibility to the spine and trims the waistline.

METHOD Sit on the floor or your yoga mat with your legs stretched out in front of you. Bend your left leg and bring your left heel in towards the groin, then bend your right knee, placing the right foot on top of the left thigh (1). If you find this uncomfortable, then place your right foot on the floor in front of the left one.

Put your right hand on the floor at the base of your spine (2) and place your left hand on your right knee (3). If the right foot is on the thigh, see if you can take your right hand behind your back to grab your right big toe (4).

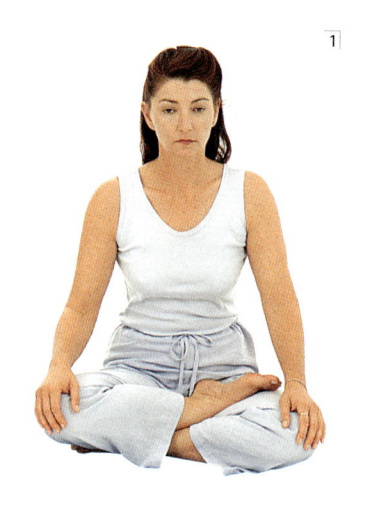

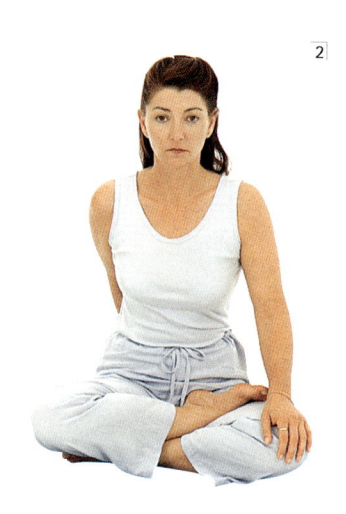

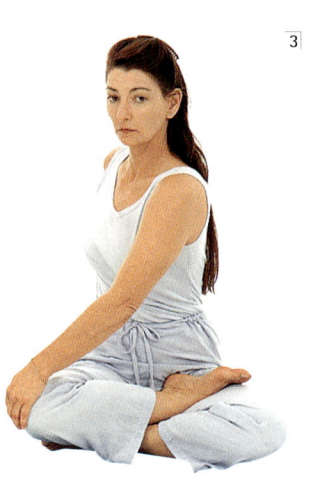

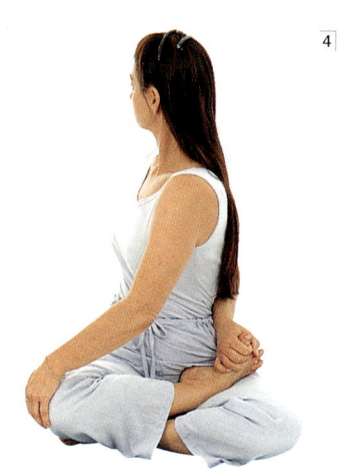

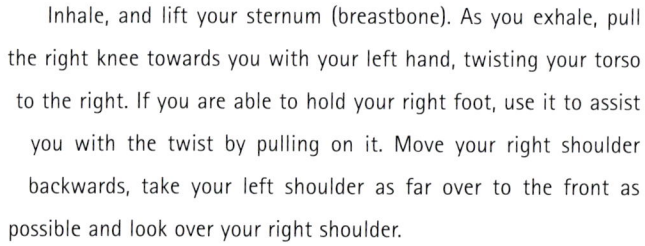

Inhale, and lift your sternum (breastbone). As you exhale, pull the right knee towards you with your left hand, twisting your torso to the right. If you are able to hold your right foot, use it to assist you with the twist by pulling on it. Move your right shoulder backwards, take your left shoulder as far over to the front as possible and look over your right shoulder.

Close your eyes, and hold the position for eight breaths. Release your hands and slowly face the front, then release your legs and shake them out. Repeat the exercise, this time bending the right leg first and twisting your body around to the left.

COUNTER-POSTURE Pose of the Child (see p40).

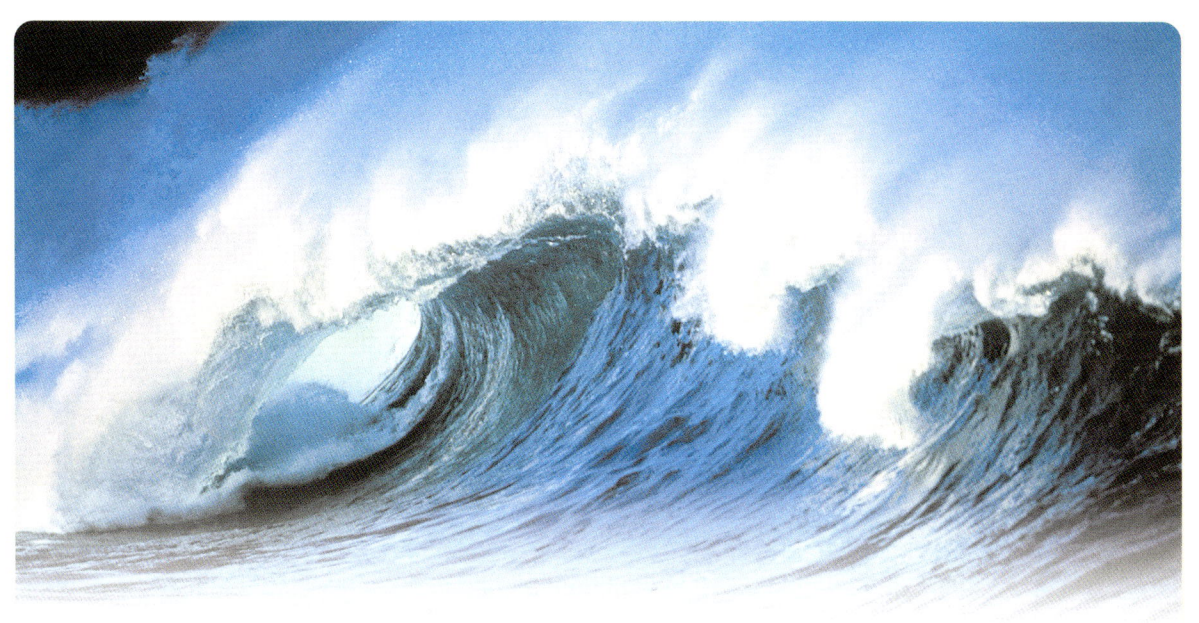

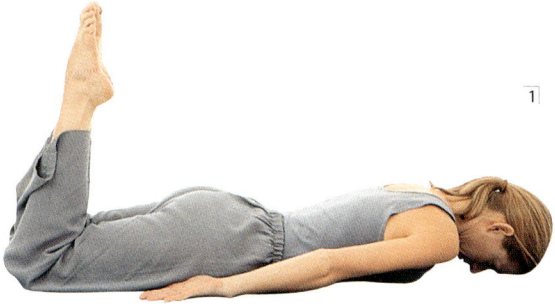

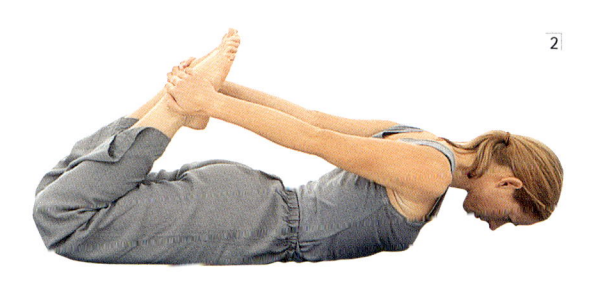

The Bow

Dhanurasana

(Intermediate)

BENEFITS This body-curving posture brings suppleness to the spine. It opens the chest and stretches the shoulders and the quadriceps (frontal thigh muscles). It flushes the kidneys and works the adrenal glands and is therefore energizing.

CAUTIONS Take care if you have problems with your spine or lower back, or if you underwent a Caesarean (C-section) and still have a tender abdomen.

METHOD Lie on your stomach and bend your knees, lifting your feet towards your buttocks (1). Reach back with your hands and take hold of your ankles (2). Inhale, and as you exhale move your feet away from your buttocks, raising your chest and bringing your head up so that you look forward (3). Keep your arms straight. Hold the posture for six breaths and then release your feet, lowering your sternum (breastbone) to the floor. If you are feeling fit and strong, then try rocking in this posture. Repeat the posture two or three times.

COUNTER-POSTURE Apanasana (see p39).

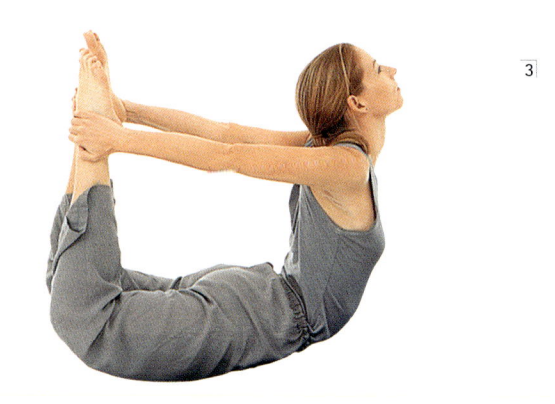

Postnatal Postures

Upward-facing Dog Stretch
Urdhva Mukha Svanasana
(Intermediate)

BENEFITS Brings suppleness to the spine, strengthens the arms, flushes the kidneys and works the adrenal glands. This is an energizing posture.

CAUTIONS It is essential that the knees and buttock muscles are pulled tight to protect the lower back. If you have lower back problems, move your feet hip distance apart.

METHOD Lie flat on the floor on your stomach with your face down and your feet together. Place your hands next to your breasts with the fingers spread wide apart and the middle fingers parallel to each other. Curl your toes under so that your feet are perpendicular to the floor (1). Tighten your knees and buttock muscles and keep them tight throughout the posture. Inhale and raise your head (2), then straighten your arms, lifting your body off the floor (3). Only your hands and the balls of the feet should be on the floor. Keep your hips dropped so that there is a small backbend. Ensure that you do not pull your shoulders up underneath your ears.

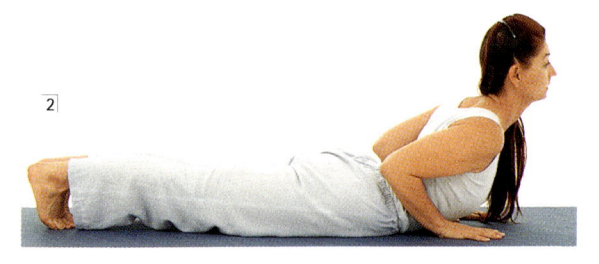

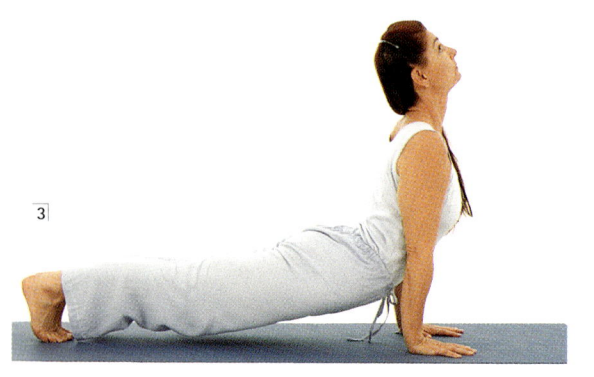

Hold the posture for as long as it remains comfortable, while breathing normally, and then lower your body to the floor on an exhalation.

COUNTER-POSTURE Apanasana (see p39).

VARIATION

Upward-facing Dog Stretch moving into the Downward-facing Dog Stretch
(Intermediate)

METHOD Go into the Upward-facing Dog Stretch on an inhalation (1). As you exhale, push back on your hands and raise your buttocks so that you move slowly into the Downward-facing Dog Stretch (2) (see p73). Inhale and drop back into the Upward-facing Dog Stretch. Keep moving from the one Dog Stretch into the other as you breathe rhythmically and evenly. Keep your breathing controlled and your movements slow. This is also called the 'Liver and Spleen' because those two internal organs derive great benefits from this exercise.

COUNTER-POSTURE Rest in the Pose of the Child (see p40).

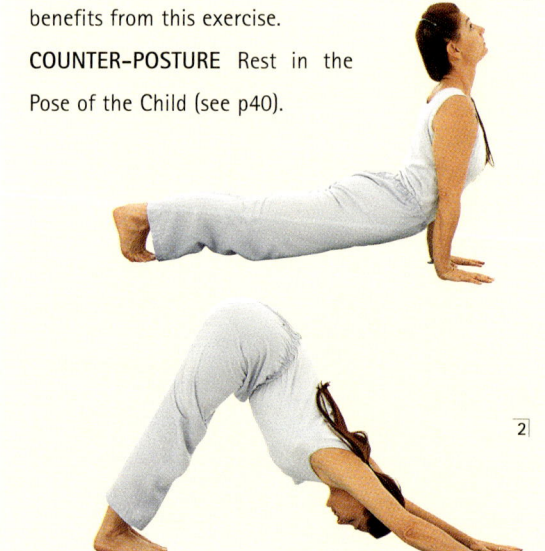

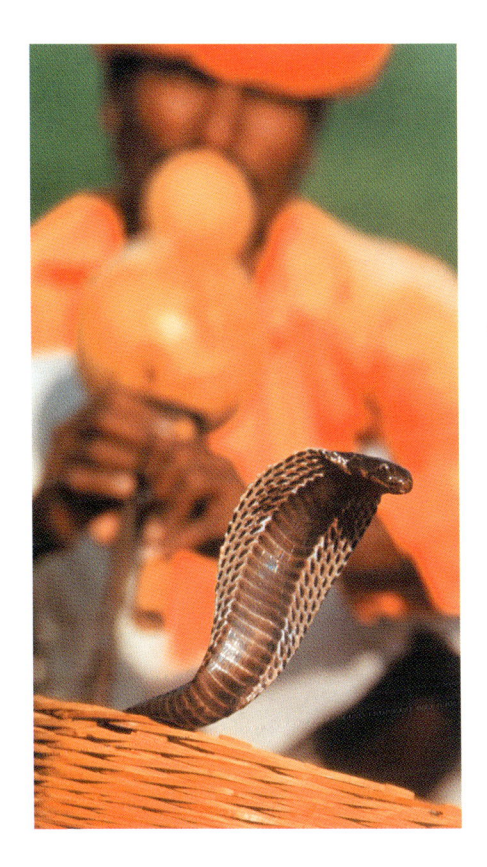

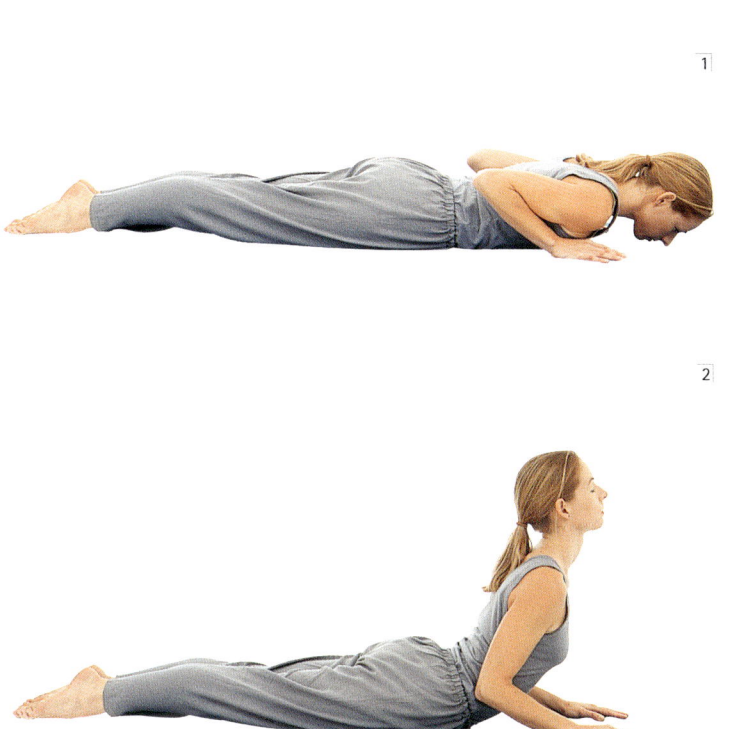

The Cobra

Bhujangasana

(Intermediate)

BENEFITS Strengthens the back muscles, improves spinal flexibility, tones the abdomen and flushes the kidneys. It works the adrenal glands and is therefore energizing.

CAUTIONS To protect the lower back, tighten your buttock muscles and pull your kneecaps up so tightly that they are off the floor. If you have lower back problems, you can still do the Cobra, but ensure that your feet are hip distance apart instead of keeping them together, as opening the legs releases pressure on the lower back.

METHOD Lie flat on your stomach with your legs straight and your nose touching the floor. Place your hands directly underneath your shoulders with the fingers spread wide and the middle fingers parallel to each other (1). Your legs should be pulled tightly together (unless you have a back problem, in which case, keep your feet hip distance apart). Tighten your knees and buttock muscles and keep them tight throughout this exercise, which requires long, controlled breathing. As you inhale, slide your nose along the floor and slowly raise your head to look straight ahead (2). Lift your shoulders off the floor so that your chest is raised. Do not straighten your elbows, keep them bent and tucked close in against your ribcage. Try to keep your shoulders relaxed, not pulled up underneath your ears.

You can do this posture dynamically, inhaling and lifting into the posture, then lowering your body on the exhalation; or statically, by going into the posture and holding it for six breaths before lowering your body on an exhalation. If you do the posture dynamically, then repeat it six times.

COUNTER-POSTURE Apanasana (see p39).

Postnatal Postures

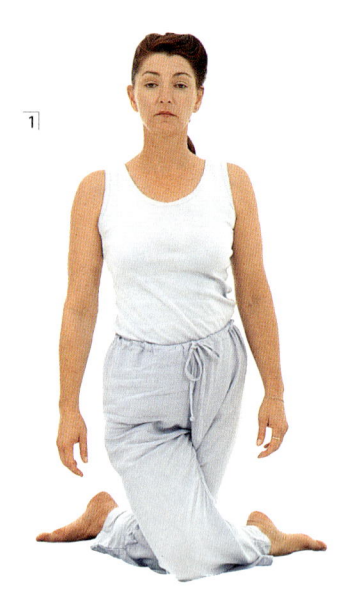

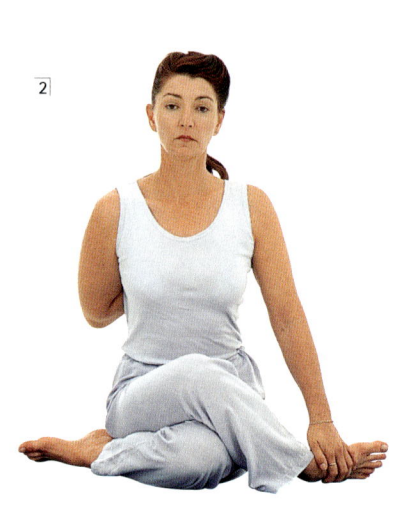

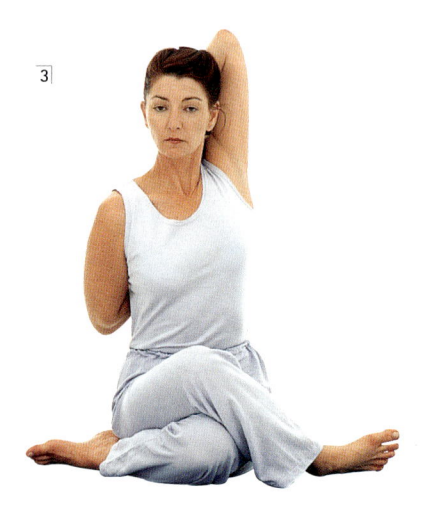

THE FACE OF THE COW

Gomukhasana

(Advanced)

BENEFITS Stretches the hips and the shoulders.

CAUTIONS This intense posture may make you aware of muscles you never knew existed.

METHOD Start in an upright kneeling position. Place your right foot on the floor in front of you and slide it around the outside of your left knee, moving the left foot to the right, so that it is out of the way (1). Sit down so that your buttocks are between your feet (2). This is a big hip stretch and you might need to place a cushion or folded blanket under your buttocks to make it less intense. Relax your hips and soften into the posture, continuing to breathe normally. Take your right arm behind your back and try to work the fingers up towards the neck area. Inhale and raise your left arm up alongside your left ear. As you exhale, drop your left hand down behind your back and grab the fingers of your right hand with the fingers of your left hand (3). Again, relax your shoulders and your hips. The more you can relax your body, the more comfortable this posture will become. Use the tips on the opposite page to help you while you are learning this pose.

If you are supple and want to intensify the stretch, then, once your hands have connected, inhale and as you exhale, stretch forward over your right knee (4). Hold for as long as it remains comfortable, then raise your right elbow and head and come back into the sitting position.

To come out of the posture, release your arms, unlock your legs and give them a good shake. Repeat on the opposite side.

COUNTER-POSTURE The Pose of the Child (see p40).

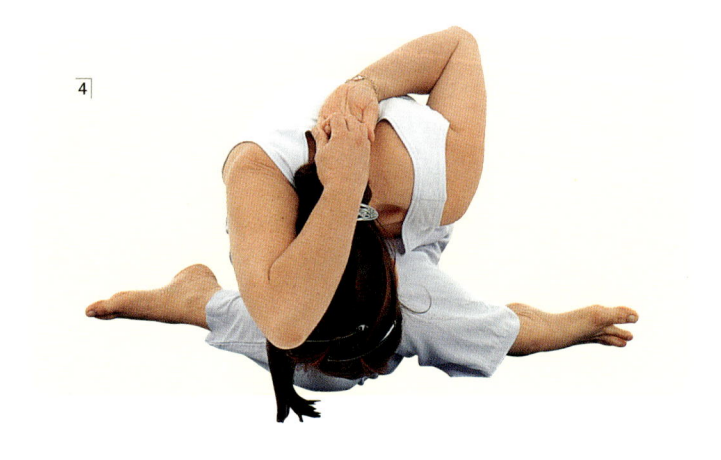

The Locust

TIP: If the stretch in your hips is too intense, then place a wooden block, cushion or folded blanket under your buttocks.

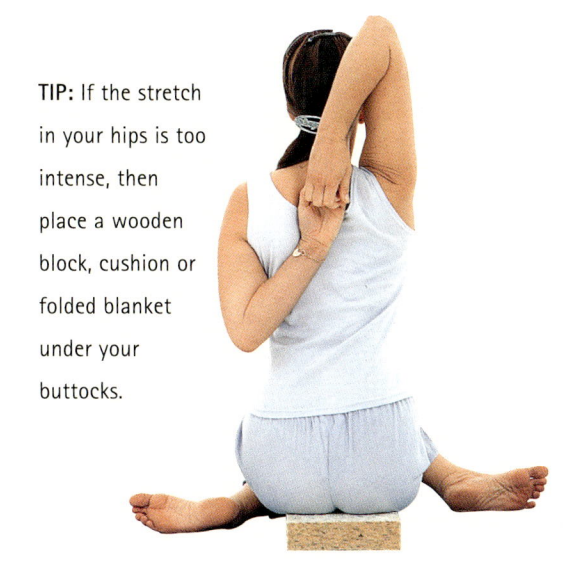

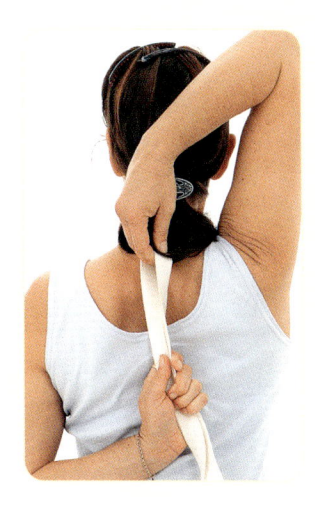

TIP: If you find that you cannot grasp your fingers behind your back, then use a belt or strap to assist you.

The Locust

Salabasana

(Intermediate)

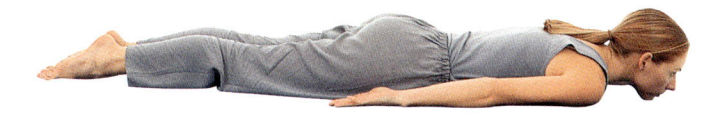

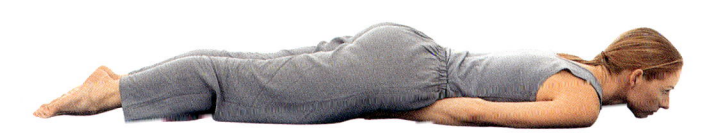

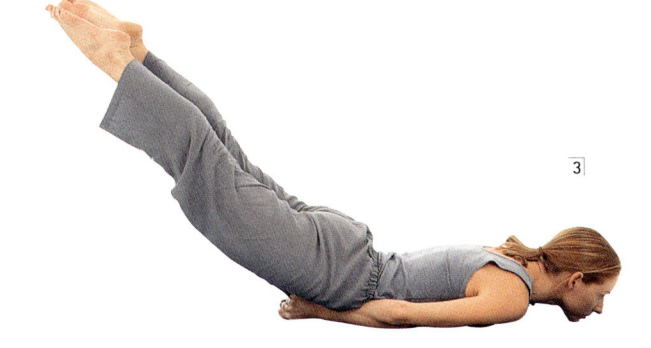

BENEFITS This is a strong posture that strengthens the lower back and works the kidneys and adrenal glands.

CAUTIONS Keep your buttock muscles firmly clenched throughout the entire exercise. If you have a back problem, keep your feet hip distance apart to release pressure from the lower back. Take care if you underwent a Caesarean (C-section) and still have a tender abdomen.

METHOD Lie face down on your mat with your forehead or chin touching the floor (1). Press your legs firmly together (unless you suffer from a lower back problem). Make fists with your hands and place them underneath your hips (2). Inhale, tighten your buttock muscles and lift your feet and legs as high off the floor as possible (3). Hold the posture while maintaining a steady breathing rhythm. When you have had enough, lower your legs to the floor on an exhalation.

COUNTER-POSTURE Apanasana (see p39).

Planning your own yoga sessions

We have prepared three complete prenatal yoga sessions for you to follow at home. To derive maximum benefit, you should do the exercises in the sequence in which they are laid out, together with the recommended counter-position for each posture (refer to the relevant page).

In addition to the sequences given here, you can make up your own yoga sessions. Start with easy postures, as this allows your muscles time to warm up slowly, and work gradually towards the more strenuous postures. Complete any sitting postures before doing standing or kneeling postures, so that you are not jumping up and down like a yo-yo on a string. Remember never to do a spinal twist after a back bend. It is beneficial to end with an inversion.

Finish each session with 15 minutes of relaxation in the Pose of the Corpse (see p26). Play some soft gentle music and practise Ujjayi breathing while you relax.

Be creative in your yoga practice and enjoy it, but at all times, observe the cautions related to pregnancy.

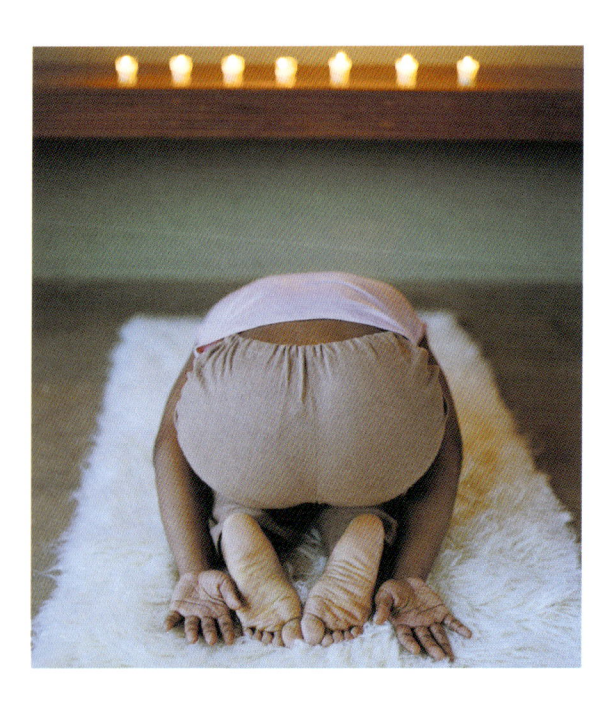

First prepared session

1 Shoulder rolls – p39

2 Hip stretches: Frog (*Mandukasana*) – p40 or the Comfortable Position (*Sidhasana*) – p41

3 Cobbler's Pose (*Baddha Konasana*) – p42

4 The Bridge (*Setu Bandhasana*) – p48

5 The Baby – p44

6 Lunges and Leg stretches – p54

7 The Crescent Moon (*Chandrasana*) – p56

8 Head to Knee Posture (*Janu Sirsasana*) – p51

9 The Mountain (*Tadasana*) – p60

10 The Tree (*Vrksasana*) – p61

11 The Dancer (*Natarajasana*) – p62

12 Squats (*Utkatasana*) – p66

13 The Warrior No.1 (*Virabhadrasana*) – p62

14 Downward-facing Dog Stretch (*Adho Mukha Svanasana*) – p73

15 Pose of the Child (*Balasana*) – p40

16 Pose of the Corpse (*Savasana*) – p26.

Second Prepared Session

1 Neck releases – p38

2 Shoulder rolls – p39

3 Cat Stretch (*Bidalasana*) – p46

4 Downward-facing Dog Stretch (*Adho Mukha Svanasana*) – p73

5 Dynamic movement: Cat Stretch (p46) moving into Downward-facing Dog Stretch (p73)

6 Pose of the Child (*Balasana*) – p40

7 The Mountain (*Tadasana*) – p60

8 The Extended Triangle (*Trikonasana*) – p67

9 Squats (*Utkatasana*) – p66

10 The Warrior No. 2 (*Virabhadrasana*) – p64

11 The Little Headstand (*Salamba Sirsasana*) – p77

12 Open Leg Forward Bend (*Upavistha Konasana*) – p53

13 The Hero (*Virasana*) – p45

14 Pose of the Corpse (*Savasana*) – p26.

Third Prepared Session

1 Upright Standing Posture (*Samasthiti*) – p60

2 The Mountain (*Tadasana*) – p60

3 The Dancer (*Natarajasana*) – p62

4 Extended Triangle Posture (*Trikonasana*) – p67

5 The Frog (*Mandukasana*) – p40

6 Downward-facing Dog Stretch (*Adho Mukha Svanasana*) – p73

7 Pose of the Child (*Balasana*) – p40

8 The Baby – p44

9 The Cobbler's Pose (*Baddha Konasana*) – p42

10 The Bridge (*Setu Bandhasana*) – p48

11 The Shoulder Stand (*Sarvangasana*) – p74

12 The Plough (*Halasana*) – p76

13 The Fish (*Matsyasana*) – p57

14 Pose of the Corpse (*Savasana*) – p26.

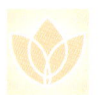

Contacts

The information provided below was correct at the time of going to print.

UK
TRIYOGA
6 Erskine Road, Primrose Hill,
London NW 3 3DJ.
Tel: +44 207 483-3344
Fax: +44 207 483-3346
E-mail: info@triyoga.co.uk

SIVANANDA YOGA VEDANTA CENTRES
Some of the over 70 Sivananda Yoga Centres worldwide are listed below.

UK
SIVANANDA YOGA VEDANTA CENTRE
51 Felsham Road, London SW15 1AZ.
Tel: +44 (20) 8780-0160
Fax: +44 (20) 8780-0128
E-mail: London@sivananda.org

USA – NEW YORK
SIVANANDA ASHRAM YOGA RANCH
PO Box 195, Budd Road
Woodbourne, New York 12788
Tel: +91 (845) 436-6492
Fax: +91 (845) 434-1032
E-mail: YogaRanch@sivananda.org

SAN FRANCISCO
SIVANANDA YOGA VEDANTA CENTRE
1200 Arguello Blvd.
San Francisco, CA 94122
Tel: +91 (415) 681-2731
Fax: +91 (415) 681-5162
E-mail: SanFrancisco@sivananda.org

GERMANY
SIVANANDA YOGA VEDANTA ZENTRUM
Schmiljanstr. 24 (Gartenhaus)
U9 Friedrich-Wilhelm-Platz
12161 Berlin
Tel: +49 (30) 859-99799
Fax: +49 (30) 859-99797
E-mail: Berlin@sivananda.org

FRANCE
CENTRE DE YOGA SIVANANDA
123 Bd. de Sebastopol
75002 Paris
Tel: +33 (1) 40 26 77 49
Fax: +33 (1) 42 33 51 97
E-mail: Paris@sivananda.org

DIRECTORY OF SIVANANDA CENTRES
www.sivananda.org
India: YogaIndia@sivananda.org
India: Delhi@sivananda.org
Austria: Vienna@sivananda.org
Spain: Madrid@sivananda.org
Switzerland: Geneva@sivananda.org
USA: LosAngeles@sivananda.org
USA: Chicago@sivananda.org

SOUTH AFRICA
ANANDA KUTIR ASHRAMA
24 Sprigg Road, Rondebosch East
Cape Town 7780
Tel/Fax: +27 (21) 696-1821
E-mail: akya@iafrica.com

NEW ZEALAND
AUCKLAND YOGA ACADEMY
190 Federal St., Central City
Auckland
Tel: +64 (9) 357-0750
Fax: +64 (9) 357-0191
E-mail: yoga@yoga.co.nz
Website: www.yoga.co.nz

AUSTRALIA
QI YOGA
53 The Corso
PO Box 1138
Manly 2095
Tel: +61 (2) 9976-6880
Fax: +61 (2) 9976-6990
E-mail: yoga@qiyoga.net
Website: www.qiyoga.net

ASHTANGA YOGA CENTRES
Website: www.Ashtanga.com

IYENGAR YOGA CENTRES
Website: www.IyengarYoga.com

KUNDALINDI YOGA CENTRES
Website: www.Kundalindiyoga.com

INTERNATIONAL YOGA TEACHERS' ASSOCIATION INC.
E-mail: info@iyta.org.au
Website: www.iyta.org.au

INDEX

alternate nostril breathing
 (*Nadi Sodhana*) 24
Apanasana 39
asanas 10
Baby 44
backbends 15
blood pressure 12, 20, 36, 58
blood volume 12
body changes in pregnancy 12, 13
Bow (*Dhanurasana*) 87
breath control 15, 17
breathing 10, 20, 21, 22-23, 24
Bridge (*Setu Bandhasana*) 15, 48-49
Butterfly Pose (see Cobbler's Pose)
Buttock Balance (*Navasana*) 83
Candle 84
Cat Stretch (*Bidalasana*)17, 46-47
chakras 15, 36, 70
chanting 25
Cobbler's Pose (*Baddha
 Konasana*) 17, 42
Cobra (*Bhujangasana*) 89
Comfortable Position (*Sidhasana*) 41
counter-postures 30
Crescent Moon (*Chandrasana*) 56
Curl Ups 82
Dancer (*Natarajasana*) 62
Downward-facing Dog Stretch (*Adho
 Mukha Svanasana*) 73
endocrine system 14
energy centres (see chakras)
Extended Triangle (*Trikonasana*) 67
Face of the Cow

(*Gomukhasana*) 90-91
Fish (*Matsyasana*) 57
Fountain (*Viparita Karani*) 12, 72
Frog (*Mandukasana*) 40
getting up off the floor 31
Head to Knee (*Janu Sirsasana*) 51
Headstand (*Sirsasana*) 14, 78-79
heart condition 36, 58
Hero (*Virasana*) 45
hormones 12, 14-15
Inverted postures 70-79
labour 16-17, 35
Leg Stretches 55
Little Headstand (*Salamba
 Sirsasana*) 77
Locust (*Salabasana*) 91
Lotus (*Padmasana*) 43
Lunges 54
Monkey God Posture (see Splits)
Mountain (*Tadasana*) 60
neck releases 38
Om 10, 25
Open Leg Forward Bend (*Upavistha
 Konsasana*) 53
Pelvic Tilt 44
Pelvic Uplift (*Mula Bandha*) 41
Plough (*Halasana*)14, 15, 76
Pose of the Child (*Balasana*) 40
Pose of the Corpse (*Savasana*) 26
Postnatal Postures 80-91
Reclining Hero (*Supta Virasana*) 45
relaxation 26, 34
safety of postures 36

Salute to the Sun (*Surya Namaskar*)
 68-69
Savasana 26
shoulder rolls 39
Shoulder Stand (*Sarvangasana*) 74-75
Sideways Swing 85
Sitting Forward Bend
 (*Paschimottasana*) 52
sitting postures 36-44, 50-53, 56-57
Splits (*Hanumanasana*) 55
Squats (*Utkatasana*) 66
Staff (*Dandasana*) 50
Standing Forward Bend (*Uttanasana,
 Padahastasana*) 64-65
standing postures 58-69
Stomach Clenching 82
supine postures 36, 39, 44, 48-49
Supine Spinal Twist
 (*Parivartanasana*) 85
supported squat 17
Tree (*Vrksasana*) 61
Ujjayi breathing 23, 26, 34
Upright Spinal Twist (*Pashusana*) 86
Upright Standing Posture
 (*Samasthiti*) 60
Upward-facing Dog Stretch (*Urdhva
 Mukha Svanasana*) 88
visualization 27
Warrior No.1 (*Virabhadrasana*) 62-63
Warrior No.2 64
yoga 8, 10, 11 30-31
 at home 33, 34
 classes 32

ACKNOWLEDGEMENTS

The author would like to thank Gayle Friedman of the Sunshine Health Academy for the use of her reference library, and Vincent Barry for the loan of his computer, without which this book would not have been written.
The publishers would like to thank the yoga models, Janine Castle (who gave birth to Samuel just three weeks after completing the photo shoot), Cathy Lambley, Christelle Marais and Amber Land, as well as make-up artist Maryna Beukes. Clothing was obtained from Ibiza Designs, Cape Town.

PHOTOGRAPHIC CREDITS

All photography by Ryno Reyneke for New Holland Image Library (NHIL), with the exception of the following photographers and/or their agencies (copyright rests with these individuals and/or their agencies).

Image Bank: pp16, 18–19, 22 (right), 23, 25, 27 (below left), 32 (below), 33 (top right), 33 (below left), 70–71, 80–81, 89 (left), 92.
Mother and Baby Picture Library: pp4, 17 (below), 27 (top right), 34, 35 (centre right).
Photo Access: pp27 (centre), 32 (top), 46 (below left), 48 (top), 61, 87 (top).
Stone/Gallo Images : pp33 (below right), 72 (top).
AKG London/British Library: pp24 (below), 52 (below right), 78 (top).
Werner Forman: p10.
Ancient Art and Architecture: p50 (top right).
Struik Image Library: p53 (top).
Bridgeman/Dinodia Picture Agency: p54 (below left).
Ruger Bonsaii Gallerie/Helmut Ruger: p86 (below left).